This book is dedicated to the Father, Son, and Holy Spirit who has fully empowered me to help many to achieve optimal health and success in life. Also, to my loving parents, Joseph and Caron Chau, who have given to me everything I have in life and much, much more

Table of Contents

New research demonstrates organic healing and
cognitive enhancement that is now possible with

Foreword

Thank you for your support of *Neuro Alchemy*.
This book was written to encourage all to pursue
becoming the best version of themselves that he/she
was created to be. Striving in life often bring us into
close encounter with various obstacles and setbacks,
some of which can, unfortunately, derail what forward
progress we have already gained for our lives. Those
who have experienced striving towards new or more
challenging goals may know of just how painful it can
be to suffer setbacks, how frustrating it can be to live
with stubborn injuries, or how lengthy plateaus of
forward progress may cause us to lose us to lose much
of the critical steam, momentum, and enthusiasm that
we need to achieve the best version of ourselves. In

my life, I had experienced several serious setbacks in health and performance that had ultimately imbued in me a burning passion for seeking out all of the latest and greatest of healing technologies available in the marketplace and within the disciplines of new medical, alternative, and complementary therapeutics, so that whenever I would encounter significant challenges, seasons of great testing, or setbacks in the future, I may be able to draw from a a deep well of robust resiliency and so that I would be able to bounce back effortlessly. Becoming resilient meant for me that I needed to research and develop greater degrees of neuroplasticity, strength, agility, and confidence for the marathon of life and for continually striving foward towards new and future challenges before me. I hope those who read *Neuro Alchemy* may walk away from this book having gained a few more effective, high-tech tools for their own personal "resiliency toolbox" that he/she could use to conquer all their future challenges and develop greater confidence in one's God-given abilities to heal, thrive, re-set, re-balance, and ultimately contribute to the world.

Neuro Alchemy is a comprised of a specially curated research collection of peer-reviewed medical journals, reputable of news articles, publication from top medical schools, randomized double-blinded placebo-controlled studies, and interviews with vetted scientists from the top research institutions.

In my line of work in health care I have had the privilege to working intimately with many neurostimulation modalities and technologies in clinical practice that are now becoming prevalent and more commonplace in the therapeutics marketplace, and which I am very glad to share with you through this book. I felt that it would be important for me to not only address all of the relevant safety and efficacy questions about each of these neurostimulation technologies, but to also take this opportunity to address the larger movement of "biohacking" as an a mindset towards discovering an entirely new and improved generation of revolutionary human health and performance-enhancing modalities. I believe that the human race is very much in a "golden period" of biohacking today with new and never-before seen technologies, supplements, and robust science coming to the marketplace everyday. I incorporating over 90 peer-reviewed scientific research studies for the sake of this discussion, but have also included as much as possible, many of the personal stories and anecdotal accounts of people of those who have used these said neurostimulation and human health performance enhancing technologies with great success in their own lives.

Biohackers are those who comprise a community of health-minded individuals who have great interest for pursuing maximum optimization of their mind, body, and spirits by utilizing the latest and greatest of what science and technology have to offer. Many whom I have encountered within this growing community have also an attitude of never-ending improvement in the pursuit of balance of all of the eight areas/domains of life, which is truly, in my personal opinion, the absolute pinnacle of bio-hacking, human performance optimization, and what I would personally refer to as the most "successful" life.

Harvard University has a Center for Wellness and Health Promotion which has a beautiful "Wellbeing Framework" which can serve us well to as a reminder that ultimately, "Wellbeing is a dynamic and fluid continuum influenced by many interconnected dimensions. The challenge each of us experience is finding the balance that works throughout the many seasons of our lives. Key ingredients in this idea are appreciating the eight dimensions of wellbeing, knowing what works for you, and living with compassion and a sense of humor."

Neuro Alchemy is primarily comprised of descriptions and not so much prescriptions for the use and best utilization of these said therapeutic modalities. Four of the most well-researched and effective of these neurostimulation modalities that I have found in my years of neurophysiology/bio-hacking research are what comprises the four chapters within this book. The successes that I experienced in utilizing human health performance enhancing technologies and neurophysiology-related medical devices have given me great new confidence towards pursuing new and even greater challenges in my life and I hope that this book ultimately give you a greater confidence and tools for your toolbox for pushing new, greater challenges, and success in your lives as well.

I sincerely hope that we may all never stop striving for our God-given best and that this book can be a most "stimulating" read for all.

Semper Meliorem,

Dr. John Chau,
B.S, M.Div, D.C, CNIM

Chapter 1- Optimal health and performance through Neurostimulation

Silicon Valley and the most prestigious research agency of the US government known as DARPA got together to collaborate, resulting in a love-child called Transcranial Direct Current Stimulation (tDCS)

The Defense Advanced Research Projects Agency (DARPA) is our nation's top research agency. It has held to its singular and enduring mission for many decades, which is to make breakthrough technologies for national security. The genesis of that mission statement and of DARPA itself dates back to the launch of the Russian Space Program's Sputnik in

1957, which completely caught the US by surprise and a solemn commitment by the United States government that, from that point forward, it (DARPA) would be the initiator and not the victim of strategic technological surprises in the future. Since then, DARPA has very successfully and remarkably executed their unique agency mission to bring to fruition many remarkable advances in technology. The vast majority of the new technologies that we currently use in the USA and by the world at large had been discovered by DARPA. DARPA's research had, several times over, completely revolutionized the direction of mankind with profound discoveries of new technologies as stealth aircraft, GPS, the world wide web (the internet), and many more. [1] Many of the world's

---

[1] Agency, D. and Us, A., 2020. *About DARPA*. [online] Darpa.mil. Available at: <https://www.darpa.mil/about-us/about-darpa> [Accessed 23 April 2020].

newest technologies have all had their origins traced back to this American government agency. DARPA's advances in technology have now also, especially in the last decade, spanned into the realm of human-machine intelligence and cognitive neuroscience technologies as well. Neurostimulation is one of these technologies that was birthed at DARPA and which is now completely transforming the landscape of human intelligence and neuroplastic capabilities of the human brain into the future.

One cognitive neuroscience technology project created by DARPA scientists along with collaboration from Silicon Valley titans and our nation's elite academic institutions is called Transcranial Direct Current Stimulation (tDCS). DARPA's stated policy for hiring only the nation's top scientists to run its research programs has brought it into collaboration with Silicon Valley. This collaboration has made it possible for brain enhancing technologies to exist, but also allowed for laypersons to easily be able to purchase tDCS devices easily and, in the comfort of one's own home, to tap into increased superhuman abilities including faster skill acquisition, supercharged multi-tasking, improved memory recall, profound new athleticism, muscular power, skill attainment, accuracy, and neurophysiological endurance.

Neurostimulation was created to improve a human's neuroplasticity, to create hyper-learning possibilities, and for super-human levels of skill acquisition

As early as in 2010, the US Department of Defense, reported to the public that their Targeted Neuroplasticity Training Program from DARPA was in the process of discovering new and effective ways to activate the brain's natural process of neuroplasticity, which is the brain's ability to change, adapt, strengthen or weaken it's neural connections, and engage intelligence in any environment. To that end, neuroplasticity training is all about helping the brain to acquire skills much more efficiently and with much greater speed, in other words, to help the brain achieve hyper-learning. The US Department of Defense reported proudly of its breakthroughs in the science of neuroplasticity and hyper-learning on its DARPA agency website, stating that "... in one of the largest effects on learning yet reported ...brain imaging and stimulation studies suggest that application of tDCS ...can greatly increase learning. The methods developed here may be useful to decrease the time required to attain expertise in a variety of settings." [2]

---

[2] 2020. [online] Available at:
<https://www.defense.gov/Explore/News/Article/Article/1

Dr. Doug Weber, the lead scientist and founding member of DARPA's Biological Technologies Office, created and managed research programs to support the White House BRAIN initiative, which launched by President Obama as early as in 2013. Dr. Weber had created DARPA's HAPTIX, ElectRx, and TNT programs, which were all tasked with developing implantable, injectable, and wearable neurotechnologies that restore natural motor and sensory functions for amputees, enable novel and drug-free therapies for treating inflammatory disease, mental health disorders, promote plasticity in the brain, and to enhance the learning of complex cognitive skills. Dr. Weber's DARPA programs specifically combined basic neuroscience research with device engineering to create new knowledge and

---

164793/darpa-funds-brain-stimulation-research-to-speed-learning/> [Accessed 23 April 2020].

capabilities for restoring and enhancing physical, mental, and cognitive performance in humans.[3]

Governments and academic institutions around the world accelerating their pace of research with cognitive enhancement technologies

Elite academic research institutions both in the US and across the globe have been busily conducting tens of thousands of research studies, independently studying and publishing scientific research on Transcranial Direct Current Stimulation (tDCS) in the last decade. In a research paper called "Hacking the

---

[3] Rnel.pitt.edu. 2020. *Douglas J. Weber, Ph.D. | Rehabilitation And Neural Engineering Laboratory | University Of Pittsburgh.* [online] Available at: <http://www.rnel.pitt.edu/people/douglas-j-weber-phd> [Accessed 23 April 2020].

Brain: Dimensions of Cognitive Enhancement",
published in the journal *ACS Neuroscience* in March of
2019, scientists explained the current atmosphere of
brain hacking technology in today's world and the
accelerated pursuit to harness the new powers of this
new frontier. "An increasingly complex world exerts
increasing demands on cognitive functions—functions
that have evolved for a fundamentally different
environment. Daily life in an information society and a
post-industrial economy requires cognitive skills that
have to be acquired through slow, effortful, and
expensive processes of education and training.
Likewise, these skills can become obsolete as the
world changes ever faster or be lost by the processes
of aging. People also vary in their mental abilities,
allowing them to acquire certain skills more quickly or
slower, which may have significant effects on life
outcomes. Strategies to improve the acquisition and
maintenance of cognitive skills are thus increasingly

important on both an individual and societal level. These challenges of our times have fostered the exploration of strategies to enhance human brain function. While people have, since time immemorial, sought to improve their performance to maximize their personal power. The present era is unique in that, not only the challenges are growing rapidly and, but so are technologies that promise to meet them. Just like the hacking culture in the realm of computer software and hardware, an increasing number of individuals experiment with strategies to creatively overcome the natural limitations of human cognitive capacity—in other words, to hack brain function. [4] Biohacking is a growing community of professionals and laypersons, athletes, special operations warriors, musicians, etc. who want to be at the leading edge of

---

[4] 2020. [online] Available at: <https://www.ncbi.nlm.nih.gov/pmc/articles/PMC6429408/> [Accessed 23 April 2020].

human performance. Unfortunately, human health and performance had been inaccessible and closed off until the pandora's box of neurostimulation science had started to become opened up to discovery and utilization by DARPA and research scientists in the past decade.

On January 29, 2020, Harvard Medical School's Harvard Health started paying more attention to brain health and human performance frontiers by publishing an article on its website regarding brain health that prophesies, "Every (human) brain changes with age, and mental function changes along with it. Mental decline is common, and it's one of the most feared consequences of aging. But cognitive impairment is not inevitable. Those who are interested in health, wellness, and human performance can develop neurological 'plasticity,' or Neuroplasticity. The article goes on to encourage those who are driven in the pursuit of becoming the best versions of themselves to develop neuroplasticity because:

1. Developing neurological "plasticity" and building up a functional reserve provides a hedge against future cell loss. Any mentally-stimulating activity that you could engage in could help you to build up a functional reserve for your brain.

2. Bringing oxygen-rich blood to the region of the brain that is responsible for thought. Exercise also spurs the development of new nerve cells and increases the connections between brain cells (*synapses*). This results in brains that are

more efficient, plastic, and adaptive, which translates into better performance.[5]

The plethora of research studies contained in this first chapter will help you to discover exactly how tDCS can be the uniquely capable tool that can of help people who are interested to achieve these two critical and recommended goals from Harvard Medical School. tDCS is a powerful and vetted tool that possesses an unique ability to boost performance in one's life through achieving a new, increased neuroplasticity and by bringing more oxygen-rich blood to all the regions of your brain, in a reliable and safe manner. The last three chapters of this book will also discuss numerous scientific research studies and

---

[5] 2020. [online] Available at: <https://www.health.harvard.edu/mind-and-mood/12-ways-to-keep-your-brain-young> [Accessed 4 May 2020].

real-world accounts from patients, celebrities, and professional athletes who explain the further benefits of enhanced oxygenation and regeneration of brain cells to boost one's neuroplasiticity and thus, improved health and performance that otherwise wouldn't be possible.

Gaining a competitive advantage through achieving Neuroplasticity

More than half a century ago, having a technological edge amongst world governments necessarily meant winning the Space Race, to be the first to put a man onto the moon, and to have functional satellites in orbit over the earth. Fast-forwarding to the present day, having the technological edge amongst world powers means having control over the technologies that would allow one to have the ability to fully interface with the human brain and harness its vast capabilities, merging and enhancing it with artificial intelligence, making humans and machines alike more intelligent. In the areas of cognitive neuroscience and within the realms of health, wellness, and human performance, having an edge over the competition also means tapping into the vast abilities body's neurophysiological systems that had been previously inaccessible for all of the history of humanity until recently. Enhanced neuroplasticity, faster healing, hyper-learning, improved memory retrieval, dynamic multitasking, increased strength, power, and endurance is now a present-day reality with the neurostimulation technologies and modalities highlighted within this book.

The science of human and machine cognition is indeed advancing at a rapid rate, as evidenced by the sheer number of thousands of scientific studies being published worldwide on this subject. In some cultures in the world, there is a stronger push by society to become more intelligent or have more cognitive prowess versus others. [6] To become more competitive in the future world, governments, academic institutions, businesses, professional sports teams and militaries that are also becoming forward-looking in terms of investing heavily in the art and sciences of cognitive enhancement, interfaces, and therapeutics aimed at healing traumatic brain and spinal cord injuries as well.

---

[6] 2020. [online] Available at: <https://www.ncbi.nlm.nih.gov/pubmed/25977093> [Accessed 23 April 2020].

Peer-reviewed scientific research studies exclaim the profound efficacy, safety, and neuroplastic effects behind tDCS neurostimulation technology

In an early research study regarding tDCS published by the Harvard Graduate School of Education in the *Journal of Cognitive Neuroscience*, scientists state that, "Transcranial direct current stimulation has been shown to improve human performance on a complex verbal problem-solving task by up to 25%." [7] In 2015, a research study published in the journal *Cortex* found that tDCS increased multitasking performance in 41 human

---

[7] 2020. [online] Available at: <https://www.ncbi.nlm.nih.gov/pubmed/18855556> [Accessed 23 April 2020].

subjects tested by a full 28%. [8] The journal *Frontiers in Human Neuroscience* reported similar results in November 2016 when it was documented the story of military scientists and contractors at Wright-Patterson Air Force Base. These elite scientists who worked at the Air Force Research Laboratory used 20 Air Force pilots in one study of performance and sustainment of multi-tasking tasks. They observed that many of these pilots started slumping in their cognitive performance whenever the demands of the job became too intense. However, these scientists discovered that by utilizing tDCS electrical brain stimulation on these test pilots, that there became "a profound improvement in multitasking skills and that tDCS staved off the inevitable drop in performance that comes with the information overload of the twenty Air Force Pilots

---

[8] 2020. [online] Available at: <https://www.ncbi.nlm.nih.gov/pubmed/26073148> [Accessed 23 April 2020].

who participated in this study." [9] Interestingly enough, the scientists also included in a concluding statement that tDCS neurostimulation, as used in this study, worked twice as well and three times as long as caffeine in its cognitive-enhancing effects and did so without any detectable negative consequences to the health of these pilots.

The Journal of World Surgery also echoed similar findings regarding tDCS in their unique experiment where researchers studied twenty-two medical students who utilized tDCS in the domain of neurological surgery education. Twenty-two medical school participants were trained to acquire tumor resection skills using a virtual reality neurosurgical simulator and received either tDCS or sham (fake) tDCS over the primary motor cortex area of their

---

[9] 2020. [online] Available at: <https://www.frontiersin.org/articles/10.3389/fnhum.2016.00589/full [Accessed 23 April 2020].

brains while training with the virtual reality neurosurgical simulators. Those receiving tDCS intervention amazingly increased the amount of tumor they resected, increased the effectiveness of resection, reduced the duration of the surgery, and improved resection efficiency. No adverse events were documented, and sensation severity did not differ between stimulation groups. The scientists concluded their research with tDCS as an addition of to neurosurgical training may very well enhance skill acquisition in a simulation-based environment by as much as 30%. [10]

The benefits of utilizing tDCS for the acquisition of complex skills in the discipline of music performance were also found by the Institutes of Cognitive Neuroscience and Neurology, University

---

[10] 2020. [online] Available at: <https://www.sciencedirect.com/science/article/abs/pii/S1878875017314249> [Accessed 23 April 2020].

College London. Researchers there found that utilization of tDCS lead to a 30% increase in speed and accuracy on a piano playing task, and that tDCS augmented synergistic learning, leading to faster and more synchronized execution. This remarkable effect on the piano playing task even persisted for 4 weeks after having the tDCS neurostimulation! [11] A remarkably large and diverse collection of scientific evidence from research institutions from around the world all seem to agree in their findings that tDCS can be amazingly effective at helping to supercharge human performance in wide variety of multitasking tasks and with complex skill acquisition. The pandora's box of safe and effective cognitive enhancement, neuroplasticity, and super-human capabilities has been documented extensively and is significantly

---

[11] 2020. Available at: <https://www.ncbi.nlm.nih.gov/pubmed/24431461> [Accessed 23 April 2020].

stimulating to the growing community of world-wide biohackers and performance enhancement enthusiasts, to say the least.

Real world testing of tDCS shows people who are run faster, jump higher, lift heavier weights, and learn faster with super-human improvements. Organizations start to utilize tDCS to "stimulate" more wins and success with their teams

Hope Hodge Seck, an award-winning investigative reporter with Military.com uncovered tDCS neurostimulation technologies in testing within top-tier military special operations teams. Her article titled, "Super SEALs: Elite Units Pursue Brain-Stimulating Technologies" . Hope explained that transcranial electrical stimulation was one of the technologies that was even touted publicly by Defense Secretary Ash Carter in July 2016, as part of his Defense Innovation Unit, or "DIUx" initiative. Multiple SEAL units have begun actively testing the effectiveness of tDCS technology, in a statement from officials with Naval Special Warfare Command. "We plan on using this technology for mission enhancement," Navy SEAL Admiral Tim Szymanski went on record to state that, "The enhanced human performance piece is critical to the life of our operators". Admiral Szymanski originally had his eye on a variety of technologies to enhance training and performance in his Navy SEALs, not excluding certain pharmaceutical drugs such as Ritalin, Modafinil, and even amphetamines. These drugs had been already been extensively examined, studied, and tested with U.S. Air Force pilots for their cognitive enhancement promises, but unfortunately it was well documented that those interventions had quickly fallen out of favor largely due to their severe and long-term negative side effects. The upside to those specific pharmaceutical medications was that for a short term, attention span, concentration, and alertness all became enhanced, however, it was always quickly followed by an onslaught of negative side effects that lingered on for periods long after their use. Those profound negative side effects were ultimately the reason that military commanders stopped pursuing those pharmaceutical medications and interventions any further. They were found to be "non-supportive of the overall mission for boosting the complex cognitive processing abilities in our elite warriors". Seriously long-lasting problems with pharmaceutical interventions included addiction, negative influence on later demands for cognitive performance, decreased general alertness, and slew of multiple types of mood disorders made these pharmaceutical medications a poor candidate for optimal health and performance in the long run.

However, the positive scientific findings supporting tDCS neurostimulation quickly became the jewel of the Admiral's eye as being far more superior as a possible candidate for human performance enhancement with his men. Hope Secks relayed her personal observations with the testing of tDCS in use with the SEAL teams. She recounts that, "The elements testing this technology were Navy SEALs who were tasked with surveying, monitoring these screens ... their abilities to concentrate on the task being tested would quickly fall off in about 20 minutes. Interestingly enough, with a little bit of electrical stimulation that was applied with tDCS, and they were then able to maintain their same peak performance with a profound ability to concentrate for 20 straight hours, as opposed to only 20 minutes without tDCS on the same task!

The Silicon Valley representative that provided these tDCS headsets to the Navy SEALs for testing was Brett Wingeier, Chief Technology Officer of a company that used to be called Halo Neuroscience. His company made tDCS headsets that looked similar to and played music in the form factor of popular, modern, over-the-ear headphones. Brett Wingeier exclaimed in statements that, "Even compared with all of the athletes that this company has worked with in the past, the focus and determination of the SEALs were nothing if not impressive. They are training at these amazingly high levels, and the amount they can training that they can sustain is only limited only by things like physical recovery. For the notoriously hard-training and sleep-deprived operators such as the Navy SEALs, neurostimulation devices offer a type of greater efficiency in training, allowing special operators to ultimately train less and yet see the same results, or similarly, train at the same level, but get a larger boost in their performance and skill." [12]

Transcranial direct current stimulation technology had gone on to prove useful not only in developing explosive new mental powers for SEALS, but also for professional athletes who require powerful vertical leaps, sudden starts, and quick maneuvering. tDCS when tested, as started showing solid capabilities of helping people to vastly improve upon their highly specialized skills and tasks, such as those involved competition pistol-shooting

---

[12] 2020. Available at: <https://www.military.com/daily-news/2017/04/02/super-seals-elite-units-pursue-brain-stimulating-technologies.html> [Accessed 30 April 2020].

performance. Halo Sport, which has since gone out of business since the latest edit of this book, had tested this premise out by giving their tDCS headsets to National and World Speed Shooting Champion Max Miche, the Captain of Team Sig Sauer, along with his entire team for testing. Max Miche stated, "I've been wearing Halo Sport for the last five months. I identified a problem at one point last year where my left foot was dragging and it wasn't allowing me to be able to shoot as soon as I entered a position or maintain that balance and stability that I needed to fire at a high rate of speed. Halo Sport has provided me a platform for training at the gym to make me better at what I do on the practice field and the competition range." Similarly, Shane Coley, Captain of Team Glock shooting team, said that after wearing Halo Sport tDCS headsets, "Last year, it took me four-five months of training to feel a certain way... to feel like I was prepared to show up at a match. When we started tDCS neurostimulation along with our training, I went out to the range and I felt like I had the equivalent of three-four months of range practice. I felt like everything came back instantly. tDCS makes every second of every minute of training I get worth it and makes the most out of everything I'm able to do."

Professional athletes and sports coaches report profound improvements in cognitive abilities, athletic abilities, and also a large "competitive advantage" with tDCS utilization

When in 2015, 2017, and in 2018 the Golden State Warriors won the NBA championships, it is notable that they were actively utilizing Halo Sport's tDCS headsets during their practice sessions, and similarly, so were the UNC Tar heels when they won their NCAA championship in 2017. Was this purely coincidental, or was there a strong correlation in the increases in athletic performance and championship-level athleticism with tDCS neurostimulation?

In 2017, *Frontiers in Human Neuroscience* published an interesting research study that concluded stating that the effects of 20 min of tDCS on trained cyclists during an incremental cycling test found significantly improved peak power, as well as reduced heart rate as well as perception of effort at submaximal workloads. The researchers reported reduced perception of effort and increased endurance with 9 cyclists following tDCS anodal stimulation. Similarly, they found scientific evidence that elite athletes gained a potential competitive advantage in cognitive performance and mood elevation, with 2 mA of electric current applied at the anode over the left dorsolateral prefrontal cortex. [13]

In 2019, a scientific study that utilized tDCS in an experiment evaluating 12 experienced bodybuilders had randomly assigned these bodybuilders to receive either sham or real tDCS. The study found that regarding muscular strength, endurance, and electrical activity, one-repetition maximum (1RM), muscular endurance (SEI), and surface electromyography over quadriceps femoris muscle (sEMG) factors improved by 4.4%, 16.9%, and 5.8%, respectively. [14]

---

[13] 2020. [online] Available at: <https://www.ncbi.nlm.nih.gov/pmc/articles/PMC5423975/> [Accessed 13 May 2020].

[14] 2020. [online] Available at: <https://www.ncbi.nlm.nih.gov/pmc/articles/PMC6675286/> [Accessed 13 May 2020].

In a research study published in the *Journal of NeuroEngineering and Rehabilitation* in 2019, the researchers in that study concluded, "There is increasing scientific evidence that tDCS modulates the brain to establish new patterns of activity and functional improvement in healthy as well as in disabled individuals. [15]

Another study published in the scientific journal *Frontiers in Psychiatry* in 2016 examined 10 professional athletes from three different sports(judo, swimming, and rhythmic gymnastics). They received tDCS anodal stimulation (2 mA) for 20 min on the left dorsolateral prefrontal cortex for ten consecutive weekdays. The researchers in this study concluded, "We observed a positive effect of tDCS in their cognitive performance, including a significant

---

[15] 2020. [online] Available at: <https://jneuroengrehab.biomedcentral.com/articles/10.1186/s12984-019-0581-1> [Accessed 13 May 2020].

improvement in alternated, sustained, and divided attention in their memory scores." In addition, they found that "tDCS sessions may translate into competitive advantages for professional athletes." [16]

The exciting part of neurostimulation technology is that the science is showing that tDCS also works for most casual weekend warriors, in the elderly population, and in other domains and disciplines where complex skill acquisition and performance is important, such as in music performance. Halo Sport's Brett Wingeier went on to state that in multiple lab tests and scientific studies, tDCS was found to be safe and effective for use,

---

[16] 2020. [online] Available at:
<https://www.mendeley.com/catalogue/405c172e-e1dc-3e22-9427-7c61aa7457b3/> [Accessed 13 May 2020].

studied across thousands of documented scientific research usage cases.

Safety testing of tDCS

The *Neurobiology of Aging* journal from March 2017 reported in their study regarding the elderly utilizing tDCS. Neurostimulation was used to effect better skill acquisition in older adults, and the scientists published that an improvement of motor function by 50-100% was found in their tests, concluding that tDCS can very well help to maintain the functional independence of older adults into their golden years. [17]

---

[17] 2020. [online] Available at: <https://www.sciencedirect.com/science/article/abs/pii/S0197458016302998?via%3Dihub> [Accessed 30 April 2020].

In another safety-focused research study of tDCS published in the journal *Brain Stimulation* from 2016, it was reported that the use of conventional tDCS protocols in human trials (≤40 min, ≤4 milliamperes, ≤7.2 Coulombs) had not produced any reports of serious adverse effects across 33,200 tDCS sessions and 1000 study subjects within repeated sessions of neurostimulation. The study was careful to also include a wide variety of subjects in various age categories as well, including persons from potentially vulnerable populations. [18]

[18] 2020. [online] Available at: <https://www.ncbi.nlm.nih.gov/pubmed/27372845> [Accessed 2 May 2020].

Transcranial Direct Current Stimulation studies reveal that professional musicians are reporting more efficient practice times and also more return on investment for the same amounts of practice time

Berklee College of Music is one of the most elite music colleges in the world. In the summer of 2019, they reported on their school's website that two of their students, in addition to guest participants from Stanford University and Yale University, wrote, practiced, and played music while utilizing tDCS neurostimulation technology to enhance their productivity and streamline their learning. Alyse Brown, a summer fellow who graduated from Boston Conservatory at Berklee with a bachelor's degree in music and a minor in psychology, used neurostimulation to learn guitar for the first time and said of her experience with tDCS, "I was able to face my fears and learn guitar in just eight weeks. I even performed a duet with a friend in front of 50 people at the end of the summer. I've gained so much confidence since I started practicing with Halo Sport tDCS headsets that I hope other musicians at Berklee will have the opportunity to benefit from it as well. This could be just the thing that takes musicians to the next level." Another student, Lily Dowling, a singer-songwriter currently going into her third year at Berklee College of Music, related, "I never thought I would be incorporating brain stimulation into my songwriting process, let alone see such a big difference. With the technology, I was able to quadruple the number of songs I could write per week." [19] Similarly, Daniel Auner, a professional

---

[19] 2020. [online] Available at: <https://www.berklee.edu/news/focused/ice/berklee-college-music-and-halo-neuroscience-announce-

violinist from Vienna, was interviewed in a *Scienceline* article published in March 2020, about how he uses tDCS to help him practice and prepare for upcoming performances. After having some initial doubts, Auner says that he now regularly relies on this technology, especially whenever he feels that he is short on his practice time. He says that it helps him feel not only more focused during that practice time, but that he is also "more on top of his playing" during concerts. He remarked that he thinks the technology, which effectively reinforces muscle memory that a person is already developing with practice, is especially well suited for the practicing of musical instruments. Allowing him the ability for "being strategic in his

---

collaboration-accelerate-music> [Accessed 30 April 2020].

practicing" is one reason why Auner thinks tDCS works especially well for him. [20]

[20] 2020. [online] Available at: <https://scienceline.org/2020/03/just-because-you-can-stimulate-your-brain-with-these-headphones-doesnt-mean-you-should/> [Accessed 30 April 2020].

How exactly does Transcranial Direct Current Stimulation work on the human brain to improve upon a person's entire neurophysiology?

Dr. Praveen Pilly, who works at DARPA's HRL laboratories hypothesized, "We believe that neurostimulation boosts the release of neurotransmitters such as acetylcholine, norepinephrine, and others that play a role in modulating cognitive processes related to learning whenever a small amount of current is applied to the motor cortex of the brain. Observations on increased learning and speed of learning, often called "neuroplasticity", was effected by the modulation of increased and improved connectivity between brain areas, and not so much with the rate at which neurons fired. The improved long-range connectivity between brain areas such was observed whenever high-frequency Gamma brain waves were induced, such as when tDCS is utilized. Conversely, reduction of connectivity in the low-frequency bands were the determining factors from our study that could explain the learning improvements in humans. It is specifically with inter-areal coherence within Gamma frequencies that has the greatest link to cognitive behavioral improvements seen with tDCS utilization. Dr. Pilly, along with his HRL Laboratories researchers, have gone on to determine that "non-invasive transcranial direct current stimulation (tDCS) could increase the performance of associative learning. For example, whenever the researchers applied tDCS to the prefrontal cortex of the brain, they found that the tDCS stimulation affected a wide portion of the subject's entire brain, causing changes in functional connectivity between multiple brain areas, which then also accounted for increased learning speed that was observed." [21]

In addition, tDCS increases "neural excitability," and it does so by modulating the timing of ongoing spiking activity instead of controlling the generation of action potentials. tDCS sharply decreased coherence only at lower frequencies, with significant decreases being observed in alpha and theta EEG frequency bands. At the same time, coherence increased at the higher Gamma brain wave frequencies. These results show that high-gamma inter-areal coherence was the best predictor of learning efficiency. Finally, astrocytes are also thought to play a role in regulating neuronal synchrony. Since astrocytes are particularly susceptible to electrical

---

[21] 2020. [online] Available at: <https://www.hrl.com/news/2017/10/12/hrl-and-mcgill-scientists-confirm-transcranial-stimulation-effects-and-determine-a-key-mechanism> [Accessed 5 May 2020].

fields and synchronously release calcium in response to tDCS, they may provide another indirect pathway through which tDCS coordinates widespread neural activity. The more widespread effects are manifested as a decrease in low-frequency coherence between distant cortical sites, along with an increase in high-frequency (gamma-band) coherence between the same sites. Of these effects, the last was most strongly correlated with the animals' behavioral performance, suggesting that, for certain tasks, the beneficial effects of tDCS arise from increased communication and altered functional connectivity between distant brain regions. These findings suggest that "tDCS may be a safe, low-cost, and effective therapy for disorders in which long-range neural communication was perturbed, as in schizophrenia, traumatic brain injury, and other diseases, or even to enhance the cognitive performance amongst healthy individuals." [22]

Why stimulate over the pre-frontal cortex of the brain?

The prefrontal cortex is the portion of the brain is connected to almost all the other cortical areas of the brain and stimulating it with tDCS has widespread effects across all of the categories of cognition. Science has already shown that the prefrontal cortex is the portion of the brain that plays a vital role in emotion and mood regulation. Hemispheric asymmetries in prefrontal activity are thought to contribute to emotional processing and dysfunctions in these networks are related to mood

---

[22] 2020. [online] Available at: <https://www.cell.com/current-biology/fulltext/S0960-9822 (17)31185-5> [Accessed 5 May 2020].

disorders like depression and bipolar disorder. Higher levels of left frontal activity are correlated with more motivation and positive mood, whereas higher levels of right frontal activity are associated with more withdrawal motivation, negative mood, and increased risk for anxiety and depression. [23]

The left rostro-lateral prefrontal cortex is important for high-level processing and thought, including monitoring and integrating information processed in other areas of the brain. This area is located behind the left side of the forehead, between the eyebrow and the hairline. tDCS can work as a stimulant or an inhibitor of cerebral activity, depending on the hemispheres that are being targeted and affected by the electric current of 2 mA,

---

[23] 2020. [online] Available at: <https://www.frontiersin.org/articles/10.3389/fnhum.2020.00052/full> [Accessed 30 April 2020].

the level at which most guidelines and most manufacturers of tDCS headsets have the headsets set to stimulate at. It should be noted that tDCS headsets are broad in its actual electric current stimulation target area, largely due to the effect of "current spread" which generally covers both the areas of the brain where the primary motor cortex and the pre-frontal cortex are found.

Memories Retrieved with tDCS

"We found dramatically improved memory performance when we increased the excitability of this prefrontal cortex region," said Dr. Jesse Rissman, a UCLA assistant professor of psychology, psychiatry, and bio behavioral sciences, this study's senior author. "We didn't expect that the application of a weak electrical brain stimulation would magically make the subjects' memories perfect, but the fact that their memory performances' increased as much as it did is surprising, and it's an encouraging sign that this could potentially be used to help people retrieve memories. We think this brain area is particularly important in accessing knowledge that you formed in the past and in making decisions about it," said Rissman, who also is a member of the UCLA Brain Research Institute. [24]

Dr. Praveen Pilly goes on to amplify UCLA's Brain Research Institute's finding with a call for action for medical clinicians to help retrieve people's memories. In his statement he clarified that, "Making people smarter is not the sole purpose of this research. It is also a potentially more immediate application of DARPA's brain device for the treatment

---

[24] 2020. [online] Available at: https://neurosciencenews.com/memory-brain-stimulation-14137/?utm_campaign=Feed%3A+neuroscience-rss-feeds-neuroscience-news+%28Neuroscience+News+Updates%29&utm_medium=feed&utm_source=feedburner

of people suffering from neural degeneration that causes a loss of memory function. DARPA's Restoring Active Memory (RAM) program focuses on healing traumatic brain injury that results in a person being unable to retrieve memories. DARPA is looking to speed up the development of technologies such as tDCS that allow scientists to help those affected by this by developing new neuroprosthetics to bridge gaps in the injured brain."

Medical Spa Resorts get into tDCS neurostimulation game to help celebrities and CEOs recharge

Sha Wellness Clinic is embracing neurostimulation of various sorts, located along Spain's Mediterranean coastline in the province of Alicante, it is a luxurious and picturesque destination, and it's one of the few places in the world that offers two particular brain treatments to paying guests: brain photobiomodulation and transcranial current stimulation treatment, according to a CNBC article published on Oct 3, 2019 Sha Wellness Clinic's Vice president, Alejandro Bataller, says that the treatments attract many of the world's decision-makers and people who live very "stressful lives" to help them boost their brain activity and up their productivity at work. It appeals to guests who want their brain to function at its maximum, and for those looking to improve their energy and performance," he says.

Sha offers 12 health programs with brain treatments included in its "Healthy Aging" program, and the treatments are not cheap: Programs that include the brain treatments at the fancy resort-style clinic start at $4,000, and accommodations (for a minimum weeklong stay) range from $360 to $8,200 a night. Since adding the brain health treatments, Bataller says the clinic, which opened in 2008, has seen a remarkable increase in guests coming specifically for these treatments. Bataller, however, would not disclose how many people have gotten the brain treatments over the last year but did say that more than 50,000 people from all over the world have visited the spa, including CEOs. [25]

[25] 2020. [online] Available at: <https://www.cnbc.com/2019/10/03/sha-wellness-clinics-controversial-performance-boosting-treatments.html> [Accessed 22 May 2020].

Recreate the profound benefits of a lifetime of meditation with tDCS neurostimulation!

In a now-famous scientific research study published in 2004 entitled, "Long-term meditators self-induce high-amplitude gamma synchrony during mental practice", lifelong Buddhist meditation practitioners who had undergone meditative mental training of the Tibetan Nyingmapa and Kagyupa traditions for over 10,000 to 50,000 hours across periods ranging from 15 to 40 years, had their brainwaves recorded by Dr. Richard Davidson and his University of Wisconsin team using EEG machines. Th experiment to understand the remarkable brain waves was set up as many research studies are. A control group of student subjects who had no previous meditative experience but had declared an interest underwent meditative training for 1 week before had their brain waves recorded utilizing EEG to serve as a data from "novice meditators". During each meditative session, a 30-s block of resting activity and a 60-s block of meditation were collected four times sequentially. The subjects were all verbally instructed to begin the meditation and meditated at least 20s before the start of the meditation block. They focused here on generating a state of "unconditional loving-kindness and compassion" during these sessions. During the EEG data collection period, both the control and long-term practitioner groups tried to generate this nonreferential state of loving-kindness and compassion as meditation. During the neutral states, all of the subjects were asked to be in a nonmeditative, relaxed state. As a control, the student volunteers with no previous meditation experience were also tested after one week of training. The monks and volunteers were equally fitted with a net of 256 electrical sensors.

During meditation, the scientists who recorded the EEG data found and recorded the presence of high-amplitude Gamma brain waves in the EEGs of long-time practitioners, that weren't present in the initial baseline and the beginning of meditation sessions. Fig. 1*a* provides a representative example of these raw EEG signals. An essential aspect of these gamma brain waves is that their amplitude monotonically increased over the time of the meditative practice (Fig. 1*b*).

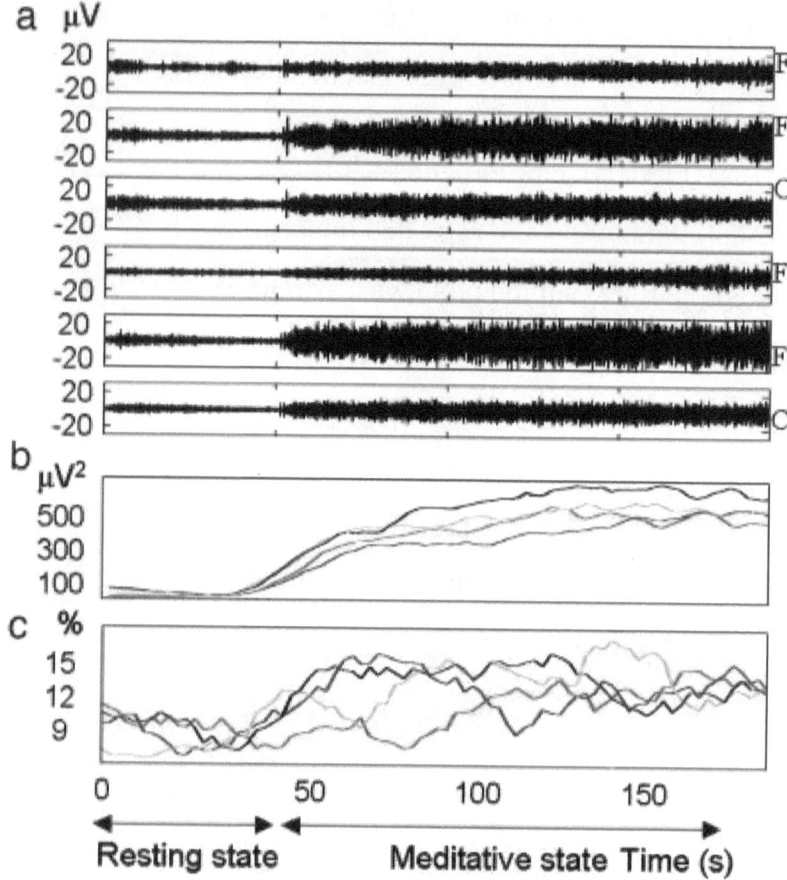

Fig. 1.

High-amplitude gamma activity during mental

training. (*a*) Raw electroencephalographic signals.

At t = 45 s, practitioner S4 started generating a state of nonreferential compassion, block 1. (*b*) Time course of gamma activity power over the electrodes displayed in *a* during four blocks computed in a 20-s sliding window every 2 s and then averaged over electrodes. (*c*) Time course of subjects' cross-hemisphere synchrony between 25 and 42 Hz. The density of long-distance synchrony above a surrogate threshold was calculated in a 20-s sliding window every 2 s for each cross-hemisphere electrode pair and was then averaged across electrode pairs (see *Methods*). Colors denote different trial blocks: blue, block 1; red, block 2; green, block 3; black, block 4.

These data sets suggest highlight the differences that the two groups had in their electrophysiological spectral profiles. In the baseline, the advanced meditators showed that their lifetime of practice with meditation was evidenced by a characteristic of a higher ratio of gamma-band oscillatory rhythm to slow oscillatory rhythms for the long-term practitioners than for the controls. This advanced group's differences were enhanced during the meditative practice and continued into the post meditative resting blocks.

The adjusted average variation in gamma activity was more than an astounding 30-fold greater among the professional meditation practitioners compared to the control group of students who had little to no experience practicing mediation. The high-amplitude gamma activity found in some of these practitioners is, to our knowledge the researchers exclaimed, some of the highest reported in scientific literature!

The scientists also concluded this particular study by stating that the findings were consistent with the idea that attention and affective processes, which gamma-band EEG synchronization may reflect, are flexible skills that can be trained (is neuroplastic). His Holiness the Dalai Lama himself was instrumental in conducting this research that was supported by the National Institute of Mental Health Mind-Body Center Grant.[26] The highest level of meditations saw some of the highest levels of gamma frequency brain waves. This causation revealed reasons behind why tDCS neurostimulation has such profound beneficial effects with it's users.

With EEG recording, electrical activity emanating from the brain is displayed in the form of brainwaves with various frequencies. Usually, transmission of messages amongst neurons in the

---

[26] 2020. [online] Available at: <https://www.ncbi.nlm.nih.gov/pmc/articles/PMC526201 /> [Accessed 30 April 2020].

brain are seen as extremely low voltages on EEG readings. Most conscious activity in the cortex of the brain produces beta waves at 13 to 30 hertz or cycles per second. More intense gamma waves (30 to 60 or even 90 Hz) are generally the mark of more complex brain operations such as memory storage, sharp concentration, and synchronization with the other interconnected portions of the brain. tDCS has been shown to be a completely novel technology in it's unique ability to induce enhancement of high-frequency Gamma brain wave coherence. What this means is that the brain is tapping into a higher state of functioning, increased processing capacity, increased brain interconnectedness, and increased neuroplasticity whenever high-frequency gamma brain wave oscillations and especially gamma brain wave synchronization occur. It is also notable to highlight the fact that these are the types of brain waves that can usually only be recorded in with brains of highly-trained musicians and advanced practice meditators such as Tibetan monks who practice meditation full-time for decades. Superior gamma brain wave synchrony can be found while recording the EEG brain waves of high-level musicians while they are listening to music—an example of a form of calm but intense focus. This larger incidence of high-frequency gamma brain wave synchrony, aka cognitive coherence, is also associated with faster learning.

In other words, when the pre-frontal cortex of the brain is induced to higher gamma brain wave frequencies, or when synchronicity amongst gamma brain waves is induced, high-level intelligence capabilities in human subjects start to emerge. Its reported that when brain waves become more synchronous and coordinated with each other, such as that which is observed during tDCS neurostimulation use, many high-level executive functions of the mind, including decision-making, cognitive control, contextual memory retrieval, faster learning capability, and multi-tasking all see measurable improvements.

Going back to the study conducted by University of Wisconsin researchers lead by Dr. Richard Davidson, we can see as revealed by electroencephalograms (EEGs), the 10 longtime Buddhist practitioners who were highlyt advanced meditation produced gamma brain waves that were extremely high in amplitude and had long-range gamma synchrony/coordination as well. The brain waves from disparate brain regions of the brain were in near lockstep (synchronous) on EEG recordings. This would be like seeing numerous jump ropes turning precisely together in harmony! The synchrony/harmony of the monk's brain waves was sustained for remarkably long periods as well. The student groups' gamma waves were nowhere near as strong nor as synchronized. It was this unique ability of these ultra-dedicated meditation practitioners to elicit synchronized gamma brain waves that distinguished their brains from the control group, the group with little to no previous meditation practice. The takeaway from this remarkable research study was that the hallmark characteristic of the brains of the most highly practiced monks, those who had a minimum of 15 years, and up to 40 years of dedicated meditation practice, was these hallmark gamma brain wave synchronies, the same sort of pattern of gamma brain wave synchrony that has is only seen with the brain waves of highly trained musicians, and also those who utilize tDCS neurostimulation.

Its known worldwide that very high-level Buddhist monks are renowned for their incredible feats of body core temperature control through only their meditation. In addition to their unique ability to be able to induce gamma brain waves to synchrony, the high-level monks demonstrated on EEG what scientists call robust brain function, or what is normally only associated with the performance of complex cognitive tasks. Such results connote more than just spiritual harmony; they reflect the coordination and synchronization of otherwise scattered groups of neurons. Gamma synchrony is normally increased in a person who is in deep concentration or is preparing to move. A lack of gamma brain wave synchrony normally indicates discordant mental activity such as seen in schizophrenia pathology. Finally, a growing body of theories proposes that gamma synchrony helps to bind the brain's many sensory and cognitive operations into the miracle of what is called consciousness. Elite level meditation practice produces not only relaxation, but also an intense, although serene attentive state, somewhat similar to when trained musicians are listening intently to music, except this skill (on the part of the high-level monks) can also be used to control functions of the body and mind that had previously been thought of as uncontrollable with the mind, such as a person's core body temperature. [27]

Dr. Richard Davidson, the lead author of this University of Wisconsin research study also reported that increased gamma wave brain activity has a remarkable ability to redistribute gray matter within the brain, as well as the ability to reduce the decline in the loss of this extremely important gray matter altogether. The decline of gray matter, according to Dr. Davidson, normally mirrors the typical decline

---

[27] 2020. [online] Available at: <https://www.scientificamerican.com/article/zen-gamma/> [Accessed 30 April 2020].

of cognitive brain function and processing ability in humans as they age. The brain has two main layers gray matter and white matter. The layer that is critical to preserve is the gray tissue. It is the gray matter that is the command and control center of the brain where all of the nerve centers are located in the brain. White matter on the other hand, is composed mostly of only transmission facilitating sheaths known as myelin, and simply functions to connect gray matter regions of the brain together to one another.

The medical journal *Frontiers in Neuroscience* published in March 2018 that meditation was found to have multiple beneficial effects on a person's mood, consciousness, and awareness. EEG brain wave recordings of Satyananda Yoga practitioners, for example, noted that while intermediate (mean experience 4 years) meditation practitioners had increased low-frequency oscillations (theta and alpha brain waves) in the right superior frontal, right inferior frontal, and right anterior temporal lobes, it was only in the advanced/elite (mean experience of 30 years) practitioners that there was the ability to induce increases in the high-frequency brain wave bands (beta and gamma). [28]

Dr. Davidson and his brain recordings of advanced practice monks unveiled a new conversation of the distinct possibility that the brain, like the rest of the body, can be altered intentionally with healthy practices. According to a Stanford University article from 2010, it was stated that Dr. Davidson and his colleagues put forth the idea that it is quite possible that with dedicated meditation practice that induces high-frequency gamma wave brain synchronization

---

[28] 2020. [online] Available at: <https://www.frontiersin.org/articles/10.3389/fnins.2018.00178/full> [Accessed 30 April 2020].

and the benefits that follow can be obtained with practice. It was also found that meditation results in a redistribution of gray matter in the brain, and a decline in the loss of gray matter. This data certainly suggests that gamma brain wave synchrony practices such as tDCS is an extremely beneficial modality in that it may induce short-term and long-term neural changes to gray matter of the brain. These neural changes allow nerve cells to communicate and operate more effectively, thereby protecting and prolonging the vitality of the brain and several important brain functions. [29]

The next natural step in scientific research with neurostimulation may very well to be have follow up studies to confirm any long term benefits from

[29] 2020. [online] Available at: <https://hopes.stanford.edu/meditation-and-hd/#pni-top0> [Accessed 30 April 2020].

tDCS. Given tDCS's ability to induce high-frequency gamma brain wave synchrony in human brains, there may be positive correlations to intellectual quotient (IQ) increases that are measurable. The possible equivalency of tDCS neurostimulation to a life-long dedication to meditation practice is also an interesting topic to explore in future scientific research.

The Spirit of neurostimulation

Oh, how the neurons sing, like celestial choirs serenading the soul! In the grand performance of neurophysiology, the mind and body find alignment, and the spirit finds solace in the gentle embrace of balance. Through the ebb and flow of chemical currents, the soul discovers its rhythm—a dance of resilience, a testimony to the interconnectedness of mind, body, and soul. In the sanctuary of wellness, the human spirit flourishes, and the heart's melody resonates with joy and vitality. With each pulse of life, the symphony of neurophysiology weaves its magic, illuminating the path to human wellness. It is a dance of restoration, a testament to the wisdom encoded within each cell.

In the embrace of balance, wounds find solace, for the symphony of neurophysiology knows the language of healing. It is a gentle conductor, orchestrating the symphony of emotions and guiding the spirit toward serenity.

Through the artistry of neurophysiology, the mind becomes a canvas of possibilities—a landscape painted with hues of peace and resilience. It is a journey of self-discovery, of delving deep into the recesses of consciousness.

In the sanctuary of the mind, where neurons weave their tales, there blooms a celestial symphony—a dance of neurophysiology and human wellness, an artistry of harmony and grace. Embrace the dance, and let your spirit soar to the crescendo of wellness's symphony.

In the labyrinth of the mind's maze, where whispers of pain reside, there blooms a celestial symphony of healing—a dance of neurostimulation, an artistry of hope that ignites the dormant embers within. Within the delicate tides of thought, a gentle pulse stirs, reaching out like an ethereal hand to touch the depths of the soul. In the realm of neurons and synapses, a tender melody plays, resonating with the heart's unspoken desires.

A symphony of currents weaves through the tangled threads of memories, casting away the shadows of affliction. Each tender pulse, like a soft caress, cradles the wounded spirit, coaxing it to awaken from slumber. The conductor of this celestial orchestra is none other than the healer within, tapping into the boundless reservoir of inner strength. The symphony plays on, dissolving the barriers of pain and sorrow, for in this ethereal dance, there lies a key to liberation. As the currents flow, they carry away the burdens that once weighed heavy upon the soul, leaving behind the fragrance of renewal. With each pulse, the symphony crescendos, guiding the spirit toward realms unexplored. It traverses the realms of emotion, dissolving barriers, and sparking a renaissance of the heart.

So, let the currents of neurostimulation embrace you, like a warm embrace on a cold winter's night. Let it be the lighthouse in the tempest, guiding your soul through the darkest of seas. In this symphony of healing, pain finds a voice, but it is not the conductor; it is merely a player in the grand melody of life. For beyond the hurt, there lies the strength of the human spirit, ready to rise and embrace the dance of neurostimulation.

Frequenly Asked Questions (FAQs)

Transcranial Neurostimulation involves the application of electrical currents to specific areas of the brain. This non-invasive and painless procedure has garnered considerable interest in the medical, research, and bio-hacking communities due to its potential to modulate brain activity and treat various neurological and psychiatric conditions, in addition to optimizing various brain functions, eliciting higher levels of functioning, maximizing skill acquisition, and many human performance capabilities as well. Imagine having the ability to enhance your physical strength, sharpen your mental acuity, and optimize your overall performance as a human being.

What is Transcranial Alternating Current Stimulation (tACS)?

Transcranial Alternating Current Stimulation (tACS) is a form of brain stimulation that delivers alternating electrical currents to specific brain regions. The alternating current oscillates at specific frequencies, which can synchronize with and modulate the brain's natural electrical rhythms.

What is Transcranial Direct Current Stimulation (tDCS)?

Transcranial Direct Current Stimulation (tDCS) is another type of brain stimulation that involves delivering low-intensity direct electrical currents to the brain. The current flows between two electrodes placed on the scalp, thereby influencing neuronal activity in targeted brain areas.

How Do tACS and tDCS Work?

Both tACS and tDCS are believed to influence brain activity by modifying the excitability of neurons in the targeted brain regions. The alternating current in tACS can entrain neural oscillations, while the direct current in tDCS can modulate the resting membrane potential of neurons.

By influencing neural activity, tACS and tDCS have the potential to enhance cognitive functions, promote neuroplasticity, and modulate brain circuits associated with various neurological and psychiatric conditions.

How Does Transcranial Neurostimulation Work?

During a Transcranial Neurostimulation session, the electrical currents modulate the excitability of neurons in the brain. The exact mechanisms of action are still under investigation, but it is believed that the electrical stimulation can lead to changes in the brain's neuroplasticity, connectivity, and neurotransmitter release.

By stimulating specific brain areas, Transcranial Neurostimulation Therapy has the potential to regulate brain circuits and alleviate symptoms associated with various neurological and psychiatric disorders.

Applications of Transcranial Neurostimulation Therapy

Major Depressive Disorder (MDD)

Transcranial Neurostimulation Therapy has shown promising results in treating Major Depressive Disorder (MDD), especially in cases where traditional antidepressant medications have been ineffective. By targeting mood-regulating brain regions, the therapy aims to improve depressive symptoms and enhance overall well-being.

Chronic Pain Management

Chronic pain conditions, such as fibromyalgia and neuropathic pain, have also been explored as potential targets for Transcranial Neurostimulation Therapy. By modulating pain pathways in the brain, the therapy may provide relief and improve the quality of life for individuals living with chronic pain.

Neuropsychiatric Disorders

Transcranial Neurostimulation is being investigated as a potential treatment for various neuropsychiatric disorders, including anxiety disorders, obsessive-compulsive disorder (OCD), and post-traumatic stress disorder (PTSD). The therapy's ability to influence brain circuits may offer new therapeutic avenues for these conditions.

Stroke Rehabilitation

Research has shown that Transcranial Neurostimulation Therapy may have applications in stroke rehabilitation. By stimulating brain areas involved in motor control and recovery, the therapy could potentially enhance motor function and aid in the rehabilitation process after a stroke.

Cognitive Enhancement

Transcranial Neurostimulation Therapy is being explored as a means of cognitive enhancement and neuroenhancement. Researchers are investigating its potential to improve memory, attention, and cognitive performance in healthy individuals.

The Transcranial Neurostimulation session: What to Expect

A typical Transcranial Neurostimulation session is performed with electrodes placed on specific locations on the scalp, targeting the desired brain regions, generally the pre-frontal cortex. The electrodes deliver low-intensity electrical currents, and patients may experience a mild tingling sensation or a light tapping on the scalp during the stimulation.

The duration and frequency of a session

Neurostimulation Therapy may vary depending on the individual's condition and the treatment plan. The therapy is well-tolerated and does not require anesthesia, allowing patients to be awake and alert throughout the session.

Is Transcranial Neurostimulation Safe?

Transcranial Neurostimulation Therapy is considered safe when administered by trained professionals or adults using appropriate protocols. The electrical currents used are generally mild and well below the threshold that could cause any harm to the brain.

Is Transcranial Neurostimulation Therapy painful?

Transcranial Neurostimulation Therapy is generally well-tolerated and not painful. Patients may experience a mild tingling sensation or tapping on the scalp during the stimulation.

How long does a typical Transcranial Neurostimulation session last?

A typical Transcranial Neurostimulation session may last anywhere from 20 to 40 minutes, depending on the specific treatment protocol and individual needs.

Are there any side effects of Transcranial Neurostimulation Therapy?

Side effects of Transcranial Neurostimulation Therapy are generally mild and transient. These may include mild scalp discomfort or headaches, but they typically subside shortly after the session.

Can Transcranial Neurostimulation Therapy be used alongside other treatments?

Yes, Transcranial Neurostimulation Therapy can be used alongside other treatments, such as medication or psychotherapy, to complement overall treatment plans.

Conclusion

Transcranial Neurostimulation Therapy represents a groundbreaking approach to brain stimulation and holds immense potential in treating various neurological and psychiatric conditions and enhancing human potential. By modulating brain activity through electrical currents, this non-invasive and painless therapy offers new avenues for improving mental health and cognitive function. As research continues to advance in this exciting field, Transcranial Neurostimulation Therapy may revolutionize the way we approach brain disorders and enhance human brain capabilities.

Chapter 2 - Lasers and LED lights able to increase human health and health performance

New research demonstrates organic healing and cognitive enhancement that is now possible with Laser and LED lights, using technology that used to only exist in science fiction movies

Microwaves, x-rays, lasers, ultraviolet light, and infrared lights are all forms of electromagnetic radiation. They each have their uniquely beneficial characteristics as well as dangers, all depending on their specific wavelength and intensity of power. At their differing wavelengths and power intensities, these forms of light can have vastly different characteristics from healing to just plain dangerous and life-threatening.

Ultraviolet lights from the sun, for example, are an essential form of light for humans to be able to naturally produce Vitamin D3 within our bodies. We know that all plant life and nearly all organic life depend on ultraviolet light to be able to grow and thrive. On the other hand, ultraviolet light at higher intensities and duration of exposure has definitively been proven to injure human tissues, with clear evidence of causation for creating deadly melanoma cancer for human skin. X-ray is also a form of light that has proven capacity to cause cancer and death when higher accumulated dosages are allowed to bombard a human over time. So then, in what ways are ultraviolet light simultaneously beneficial ad harmful? Like all lights on the electromagnetic spectrum, many lights can be both beneficial and harmful- depending on how intense the light is, what specific wavelengths of the light is that contacts human tissue, and what amounts of time those light rays are bombarding the body (dosage) will determine how much benefit and/or damage is being done or how fast a human will die from excessive exposure.

The Star Trek television episodes from the 1960's was a world-wide sensation. In the science-fiction TV drama, there were doctors onboard intergalactic spaceships who could use their handheld light-emitting devices to quickly shine light onto a person's body parts and have rapid healing take place. That technology that had once only existed in science fiction and on TV, but now exists today, is easily available for purchase the internet, and is proven by scientific research to have profound organic healing effects on human tissues and within joints such as. The scientific community has given therapeutic healing lights and lasers the name Photobiomodulation, or PBM for short. What is it realistically shown in science that be able to do?

Photobiomodulation (PBM) increases Stem Cell Production

Multiple research studies from Harvard Medical School that are included within this chapter provide the details of how Laser/LED lights with the specific wavelengths of 650nm and Infrared(IR) laser lights at a specific wavelength of 808nm can deeply penetrate your joint tissue, such as knees and shoulders, to reduce pain, inflammation, and to stimulate mesenchymal stem cells to develop. Photobiomodulation (PBMT) from top research institutions prove that increases the production of mesenchymal stem cells which then increase bone and cartilage repair growth with brand new bone and cartilage. Even traditionally difficult-to-heal joints like knees and shoulders can be organically healed with these laser lights. Stem cells are stimulated to grow and are the key to organic healing and repair within our body. These cells can produce and reproduce whatever types of tissue that is injured or damaged, and ultimately replace the injured tissue with brand new healthy tissue! Old, beat up joints can now have new life when Laser/LED/PBMT therapy is used.

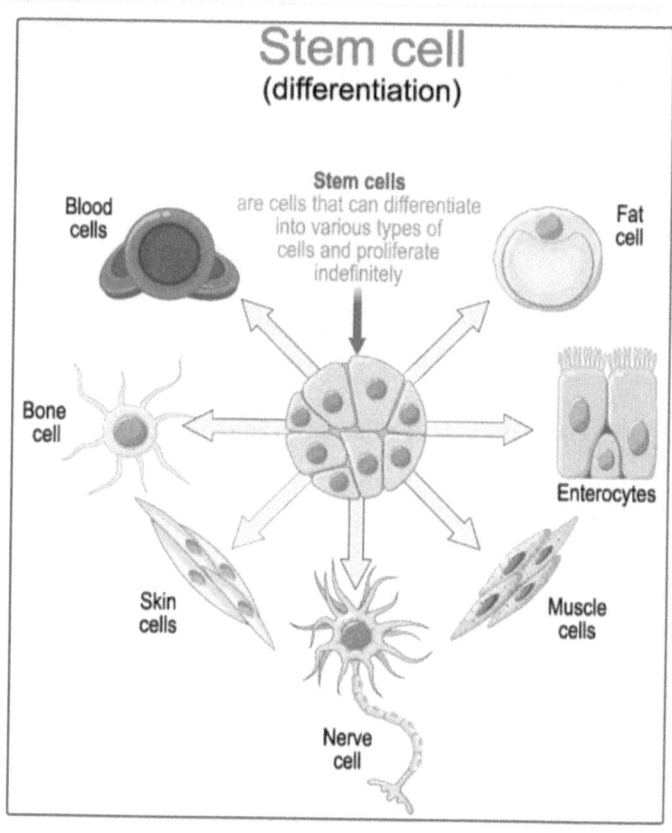

Reducing Inflammation

Dr. Hamblin from the Wellman Center for Photomedicine, Massachusetts General Hospital, Boston, MA, USA; Department of Dermatology, Harvard Medical School, Boston, MA, USA; Harvard-MIT Division of Health Sciences and Technology, Cambridge, MA show examples of that the amazing effects of PBMT that leads to decreased expression of pro-inflammatory factors such as IL-1β, IL-6, IL-10, COX-2, IFN-γ as well as increased expression of anti-inflammatory cytokines such as IL-2, IL-4, IL-13.

Blood Flow Improvement

PBMT is now proved to increase the microcirculation and perfusion of new blood flow to injured tissues via vasodilatation and angiogenesis, the formation of brand new

blood vessels!

Increase Vascular And Nerve Growth Factors

Stubborn healing by nerve cells is now a phenomenon of the past. Dr. Hamblin from Harvard Medical School has been publishing numerous studies showing how nerve growth factor (NGF) can play a role in the regeneration and growth of axonal processes to promote the survival of sensory neurons and reverse myelin degeneration. Vascular endothelial growth factor (VEGF), a potent growth factor for angiogenesis (creating new blood vessels), also plays an important role in the proliferation of Schwann cells and in the improvement of nerve repair and motor performance.

However, the difficulty in this discussion of laser and LED lights exists with explaining how therapeutic benefits can only be achieved with very specific wavelengths, intensity, pulses, and for the right amount of time (dosage). In the hands of a novice, lasers are just plain dangerous because they can easily cause tissue burns and irreversible blindness. In the hands of a trained Ophthalmic Physician, they can be extremely beneficial for laser eye surgery procedures of various sorts. The same laser lights, if dialed in at the incorrect dosages and technical settings, can bring about disastrous results such as irreversible blindness if shone into one's eyes accidently. Near Infrared (NIR) laser lights can have have incredibly beneficial effects on human heath and performance, but only at very specific wavelengths and intensities.

The same principles also apply to low-level laser therapy (LLLT), near-infrared light therapy (NILT), Red-light infrared (IR) therapy, and photobiomodulation therapy (PMBT) which are all terms describing the same therapeutic modality, the only difference being in the name. Since 2016, the US National Institutes of Health had started to favor utilizing the term Photobiomodulation" (PBM) and Photobiomodulation Therapy (PMBT) for published scientific research on this subject area. "PHOTO" means light. "BIO" means living tissue. "MODULATION" means change. Photobiomodulation is becoming popular today and is known also as red light therapeutics. Since 2016, there has been an increasingly large new library of new scientific literature from top research institutions describing the healing capabilities and also cognitive enhancement properties of photobiomodulation therapies (PBMT). Infrared saunas, for example, are now massively popular as "must-have" tool with professional athlete, bio-hackers, and health& wellness enthusiasts alike.

Nuanced conversation and detailed scientific research is included in this chapter. Dialing in the right wavelength and intensity settings on your laser can benefit your health and performance in extraordinary ways, but there are very specific dosages and precautions that are required to derive those said benefits in stimulating and/or accelerating the body's natural healing mechanisms.

PBMT for cognitive enhancement. Safety goggles are a must when working with lasers!

Photobiomodulation therapy (PBMT) using LEDs has been appearing in more and more current scientific research, demonstrating their vast capabilities to facilitate neuroregeneration, neuroplasticity, and healing in humans. The safety, convenience, and efficacy of using LEDs as a legitimate source of PBMT is published in a journal article found in *Photomedicine and Laser Surgery* in 2018. In this research study, twelve symptomatic military veterans who were diagnosed with chronic TBI >18 months post-trauma received pulsed transcranial PBMT (tPBMT) using two neoprene therapy pads containing 220 infrared and 180 red LEDs, generating a power output of 3.3 W and an average power density of 6.4 mW/cm^2 for 20 min, thrice per week over 6 weeks. Outcome measures included standardized neuropsychological test scores and qualitative and quantitative single-photon emission computed tomography (SPECT) brain imaging measures of regional cerebral blood flow. The researchers in this study concluded, "It appears the use of transcranial PBMT (tPBMT) with pulsed LEDs may improve cognitive function and decrease the regional cerebral blood flow deficits associated with chronic TBI. Considering the cost/benefit ratio and /convenience of LEDs, the economic, health, and social impact of tPBMT with LEDs in the treatment of TBI could be substantial. [30]

---

[30] 2020. [online] Available at: <https://www.liebertpub.com/doi/full/10.1089/pho.2018.4489> [Accessed 11 May 2020].

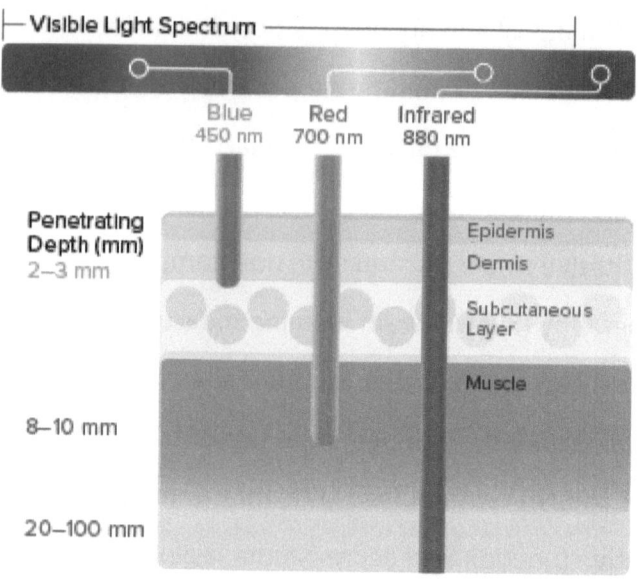

In the journal of *Neural Regeneration Research*, a research paper was published in 2016 entitled, "Multi-watt near-infrared light therapy as a neuroregenerative treatment for traumatic brain injury". It found that, "... data presented herein makes an intriguing case for the potential of multi-watt NIR laser therapy aka PBMT as a safe and effective modality for the treatment of traumatic brain injury (TBI) and possibly other neurological insults. Our data indicate that multi-Watt NIR laser therapy appears to induce a persistent change in neurological function, given patients have maintained their clinical improvements for years following treatment. Symptoms such as headache, insomnia, irritability, anxiety, depression, suicidal ideation, fatigue, and memory or concentration difficulties were resolved or greatly reduced and did not recur. Some patients are now four years since they completed treatment and they have continued to do well. Indeed, it is possible that multi-watt NILT induces a neuroregenerative change, based on the evidence of neurotrophin induction in animal models and the improvement of neurological function revealed with serial functional neuroimaging. This is a real game changer," says Dr. Henderson, M.D., Ph.D., because these patients have retained the benefits for up to four years now. For those who have been told that there is no treatment for TBI, we invite you to look closely at what we've found and you will regain hope."[31]

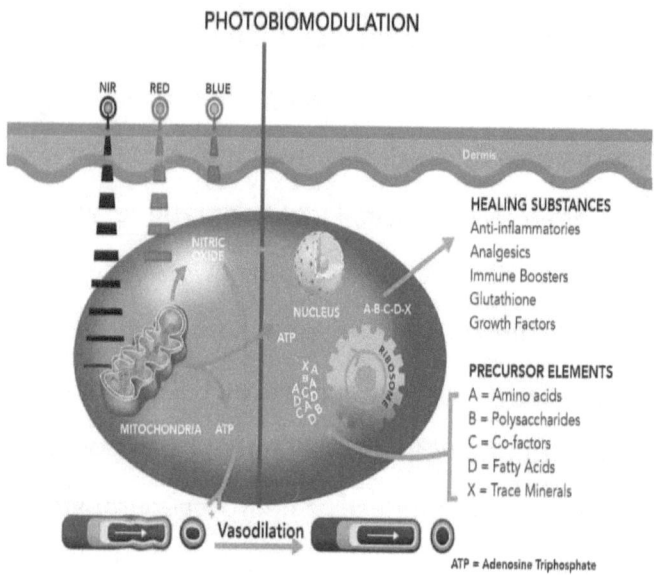

[31] 2020. [online] Available at: <https://www.ncbi.nlm.nih.gov/pmc/articles/PMC4870908/> [Accessed 8 May 2020].

In a 2015, research published in the journal *Insights in Neurosurgery* stated that scientists concluded that PMBT can modulate and control wound healing and inflammation. "Ample research is available supporting NIR light as a coadjutant therapy for various wound healing, inflammation, and pain circumstances. Advances in NIR light technology has made it more economical and much more versatile due to its compact size".[32]

[32] 2020. [online] Available at: <https://neurosurgery.imedpub.com/contributions-of-near-infrared-light-emittingdiode-in-neurosurgery.php?aid=8270> [Accessed 8 May 2020].

Past PBMT research studies were horribly done, but Harvard Medical School is leading the way now with publishing large amounts of trustworthy, positive, and gold-standard research regarding the benefits of PBMT

Several influential "systematic reviews" in the past from the Cochrane Database Organization concluded that LLLT aka PBMT, had found "no reliable evidence" for efficacy in diseases such as osteoarthritis, rheumatoid arthritis, etc. The major issues with PBMT research studies from the past involved the random use of a wide variety of different kinds of light sources, medical devices, and treatment protocols. Illumination parameters such as wavelength, fluence, power density, pulse structure, etc. had no agreement and there was no any one treatment schedule added. These factors all contributed to the poor quality of past research on PBMT. Unfortunately, variations in research study designs had led to a large number of negative trials that were published, creating much controversy on this subject at hand, despite the overwhelming number of positive clinical results that were also obtained.[33] "Many researchers fail to consider the importance of selecting the optimum parameters, nor they do not have the necessary instrumentation or trained personnel to measure them accurately, resulting in treatment failures. Another cause of failure occurs whenever the terms are misused or wrongly reported. For instance, energy (J) or energy density (J cm^{-2}) are both usually referred to as "dose," but they are, in fact, different calculations." More recently however, Photobiomodulation has made and

---

[33] 2020. [online] Available at: <https://www.ncbi.nlm.nih.gov/pmc/articles/PMC5215795/> [Accessed 8 May 2020].

is continuing to make major progress in obtaining recognition from authorities in medical schools, scholarly journals, the popular press and media, medical practitioners, therapists, and other bodies concerned with biomedical science.

Scientific literature has now improved significantly and since 2016, with reputable and comprehensive research studies regarding PBMT has been coming out of Harvard Medical School's Wellman Center for Photomedicine greatly changing the trajectory of where lasers and LED PBM therapies are headed. The lead researcher at Harvard's Wellman Center for Photomedicine, Dr. Michael Hamblin, defines Photobiomodulation (PBM) as the use of red or near-infrared light to stimulate, heal, regenerate, and protect tissue that has either been injured, is degenerating, or else is at risk of dying. He explains that there is evidence that many seemingly diverse cognitive conditions can all be beneficially affected by applying light to the head. There is even the possibility that PBM could be used for cognitive enhancement in normal healthy people he says. In this transcranial PBM (tPBM) application of lasers and LEDs, near-infrared (NIR) light is often applied to the forehead because of the better penetration through the skull to the brain (no hair, longer wavelength). Some researchers have used lasers, but recently the introduction of inexpensive light-emitting diode (LED) arrays has allowed the development of light-emitting helmets or "brain caps" as well.

Dr. Hamblin states that wavelengths in the range 600–700 nm are used to treat superficial tissue, and longer wavelengths in the range 780–950 nm, which penetrate further, are used to treat deeper-seated tissues. Wavelengths in the range 700–770 nm have been found to have limited biochemical activity and are therefore not used.

How does PBMT stimulate organic healing within human tissues exactly?

The beneficial effects of tPBM on the brain can be explained by increases in cerebral blood flow, greater oxygen availability, oxygen consumption, improved ATP production, and mitochondrial activity in the cerebral cortex. There are many reports that a brief exposure to light providing (especially in the case of experimental animals that have suffered some kind of acute injury or traumatic insult) beneficial effects lasting days, weeks, or even months, through the activation of signaling pathways and transcription factors that cause changes in protein expression. The effects of PBMT on stimulating mitochondrial activity and blood flow are by themselves very unlikely to explain the long-lasting effects of PBMT. However, recent scientific reviews listed not less than fourteen different transcription factors and signaling mediators being reported to be activated after light exposure within the human body, meaning that there are profound organic healing mechanisms that are triggered with tPBMT. [34]

Another group of researchers who have studied PBMT proposed that the mechanism of PBMT's effect could also involve the stimulation of c-kit-positive mesenchymal stem cells (MSCs) in autologous bone marrow, enhancing the capacity of MSCs to infiltrate the brain and clear out β-amyloid plaques. It appears that stem cells are particularly sensitive to light and PBMT induces stem cell activity, as shown by increased cell migration,

---

[34] 2020. [online] Available at: <https://www.ncbi.nlm.nih.gov/pmc/articles/PMC5215870/> [Accessed 20 May 2020].

differentiation, proliferation and viability, as well as by activating protein expression. Mesenchymal stem cells, usually derived from bone marrow, dental pulp, periodontal ligament, and from adipose tissue, proliferate more after light irradiation (usually with wavelengths ranging from 600 to 700 nm). It should be noted that the calvarial bone marrow of the skull contains substantial numbers of stem cells within it that respond to light exposure! Stem cell growth and proliferation means that the body is able to replace old damaged cells with new fresh cells, a normal process of healing and regeneration of the human body that typically slows down with age.

The Neural Regeneration Research journal states that PMBT has shown demonstrable neuroregeneration and repair through the mechanisms of activating anti-inflammatory processes, increase adenosine triphosphate (ATP) production, modulate reactive oxygen species, activate mitochondrial DNA replication, increase early-response genes, increase growth factor expression, induce synaptogenesis, and stimulate cell proliferation as it penetrates tissue at different depths. PMBT facilitates the release of nitric oxide supporting the body with improved circulation. [35] Improved circulation through increased blood flow is one of the most vital components of the body's healing process by bringing oxygen, nutrients, and other vital components necessary for normal functioning to that part of the body.

In a 2013 research study published in the journal *Biochemical Pharmacology*, the researchers explain that the tissue called chromophore cytochrome c oxidase (CCO) is proposed to be

---

[35] 2020. [online] Available at: <https://www.ncbi.nlm.nih.gov/pmc/articles/PMC487090 8> [Accessed 25 May 2020].

responsible for the underlying mechanism that produces the many PBMT effects. COO has absorbed bands of light energy around 665 nm and 810 nm. Cytochrome oxidase has a key role in neuronal physiology, as it serves as an interface between oxidative energy metabolism and cell survival signaling pathways. Cytochrome oxidase is an ideal target for cognitive enhancement, as its expression reflects the changes in metabolic capacity underlying higher-order brain functions. [36]

[36] 2020. [online] Available at:
<https://www.ncbi.nlm.nih.gov/pubmed/23806754>
[Accessed 8 May 2020].

Cognitive enhancement and Neuroplasticity are well-documented with PBMT, but make sure to wear goggles when handling those lasers!

In a 2017 study published in the *Journal of Neurology and Neuroscience*, transcranial sessions of near-infrared (tNIR) aka PBMT stimulation using 1060-1080 nm light-emitting diodes (LEDs) showed incredible neuroplastic effects of transcranial NIR stimulation (tNIRS) as a tool on the motor cortex to modulate cortical excitability in the corticospinal pathway and intracortical circuits. They used tNIRS at a wavelength of 810 nm for 10 min over the primary in human brains in 55 healthy volunteers. They concluded that tNIRS is suitable as a tool for influencing cortical excitability and activity. Recent human and animal studies have demonstrated the NIR light applied over the cortex has a beneficial effect on stroke rehabilitation and may minimize the cognitive deficits in traumatic brain injury. The scientists in this study concluded that "... our study showed results suggestive a trend of improvement in executive functioning; clock drawing, immediate recall, praxis memory, visual attention and task switching as well as improved EEG amplitude and connectivity measures. Neuroplasticity has also been reported with NIR light stimulation and mitochondrial enhancement.[37] Neuroplasticity had been demonstrated in this study by enhancing the body's abilities to recover from cognitive deficits and enhance cognition as

---

[37] 2020. [online] Available at: <https://www.jneuro.com/neurology-neuroscience/photobiomodulation-with-near-infrared-light-helmet-in-a-pilot-placebo-controlled-clinical-trial-in-dementia-patients-testing-memor.php?aid=18528> [Accessed 8 May 2020].

determined by established cognitive determination tests, which in turn, also translates to health and performance increases in a person's overall quality of life.

In the scientific journal, *Photomodulation, Photomedicine, and Laser Surgery*, there is an article in 2019 that is a significant review study comprised of 7 PBMT research studies that were performed on young, healthy subjects (17-35 years of age), and 2 PBMT studies that were conducted on older (≥49 years of age), healthy subjects. A meta-analysis was performed on 6 full-text publications whose subjects were young adults. The scientists concluded in their review study that PBMT demonstrates a significant, beneficial effect on the cognitive performance of young, healthy individuals.[38]

This sort of medical technology used to only exist within science fiction film, where a small hand held medical device is waved over a person's body and almost magically, there is organic healing that takes place within the human body. Now in our present day and specifically since 2016, there was been great number of scientific research coming out of elite research institutions such as from Harvard Medical School showing us the lasers and LED PBMT can be the modern, non-fiction equivalent to those medical technologies we used to only see in fantasy scenarios with handheld NIR devices that are available on the market.

---

[38] 2020. [online] Available at: <https://www.ncbi.nlm.nih.gov/pubmed/31549906> [Accessed 8 May 2020].

Cognitive enhancement of this sort may be attractive to corporate executives, athletes, elite military, weekend warriors, the elderly population, as well as health and wellness enthusiasts who may be excited to know that PBMT may be a viable, portable, and user friendly tool in the toolbox for those who seek improve their cognitive abilities and/or overcome health and performance obstacles in their lives utilizing natural non-pharmaceutical therapies.

In 2015, there was a research study conducted in conjunction with Harvard Medical School in found that a specific high-powered, near-infrared light (NIR) can effectively re-energize damaged brain cells after penetrating the skin and skull. All the patients in the study reported significant clinical improvement in their condition with no negative side effects, according to Theodore Henderson, MD, Ph.D., who co-authored the study along with Dr. Larry Morries, and Paolo Cassano of Massachusetts General. This is the second largest study of NIR for brain injury and the only one using the more powerful Class-IV laser to deliver NIR, Dr. Henderson said. The exciting news is that NIR light, in the 10-15W range at 810 nm and 980 nm, can safely and effectively treat chronic symptoms of TBI, Dr. Henderson states. [39]

Caution against the use of Class IV lasers by untrained professionals! Permanent blindness and/or tissue burns possible with certain lasers

It should be noted that Class IV level lasers, compared to Class I through III lasers, can be unnecessarily dangerous to utilize as a therapeutic

[39] 2020. [online] Available at: <https://pubmed.ncbi.nlm.nih.gov/26347062/> [Accessed 20 May 2020].

modality when used outside of the environment of a controlled medical facility. Class IV lasers are only recommended for use by trained physicians who are utilizing protective equipment for their eyes and tissues, as well as for the patient's eyes and tissues. Soft tissue burns can be imminent with Class IV lasers and are typically used for that exact purpose, as a surgical tool for burning through soft tissue.

Laser classification is determined by not just a question of optical output power, but also wavelength, a divergence of the beam, emission area, pulsing parameters, exposure rates, et cetera. Regarding Class IV high power lasers, it has not been proven in both the scientific and clinical literature that high power is better than low power, in fact, the opposite has been proven to be true! There is a therapeutic "optical" response window between 600 and 950 nm wavelength of light and a biphasic dose-response curve governed by the Arndt-Schulz law, within which the positive bioregulatory effects occur within the human body. [40]

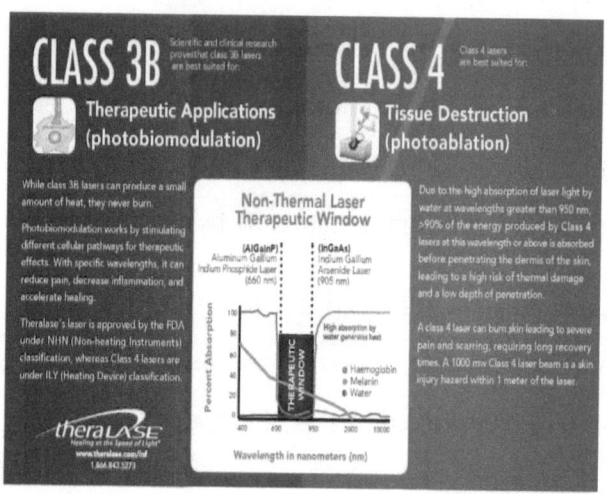

[40] 2020. [online] Available at:
<https://www.sciencedirect.com/science/article/pii/S2214647416300381> [Accessed 8 May 2020].

Dr. Lothar Lilge, Ph.D., clarifies the science of why more powerful Class IV PBMT lasers are not more beneficial than lower power lasers, and shouldn't normally be used outside of surgical environments, where cutting and burning of tissues is needed. He states that the use of Class IV lasers have a high potential of delivering non-optimal treatment doses of energy due to their lack of penetration and excessive MPE; thus presenting a greater risk of burning patients, particularly those patients with dark hair follicles. Too much power and the wrong wavelengths simply equates to the expense of more money without the requisite return in better clinical effects. Therefore lasers with output powers exceeding 500 mW are considered unnecessarily strong and downright dangerous to conduct PBMT therapeutic treatments with in the vast majority of cases, and especially by untrained individuals.

Class IV lasers have been on the market for years but have only been approved strictly for surgical applications; such as general surgery and tissue ablation for port wine stains, spider veins, et cetera. Scientific and clinical research proves that class III B lasers are best suited for therapeutic applications and class IV lasers are best suited for tissue destruction, in most cases. [41]

A few more precautionary measures for those who wish to utilize PBMT. Protect your eyes!

It is well known that photons generated by a laser using a wavelength in the near infrared range (IR-A range of 700–1400 nm), such as those used in

---

[41] 2020. [online] Available at: <https://theralase.com/everything-things-need-know-class-3-vs-class-4-lasers/> [Accessed 20 May 2020].

translational and clinical development, may cause retinal damage if the laser probe is directed toward the eye or the beam is reflected off of a surface. Other contraindications to consider include use of PBMT in people who have sustained high or low blood glucose (>300 or <60 mg/dl), sustained hypertension (systolic blood pressure >220 mmHg or diastolic blood pressure >140 mmHg) or hypotension (systolic blood pressure <80 mmHg or diastolic blood pressure <50 mmHg), history of vascular disease and use of an intravenous or intra-arterial thrombolytic. [42]

---

[42] 2020. [online] Available at: <https://www.ncbi.nlm.nih.gov/pmc/articles/PMC3270070/> [Accessed 8 May 2020].

Which specific types and dosages of Laser or LED PMBT are safe for therapeutic use?

A wide array of different light sources (lasers and LEDs) have been employed for PBMT. Infrared lights are becoming popular with professional athletes and medical clinicians for organic healing within aching joints. However, it is known that if the incorrect parameters are applied, the light treatment is likely to be ineffective. For example, there are systematic reviews and meta-analysis studies conducted of randomized, double-blind, placebo-controlled, clinical trials (RCTs) scientific literature such as from Bjordal, who identified 14 RCTs of suitable methodological quality. Unfortunately, 4 out of the 14 RCTs failed to report significant positive effects of PBMT because the irradiance was either too low, too high, or had an insufficient delivery of energy.

Another example of a systemic scientific review was performed by Tumilty of 25 RCTs of tendinopathies, 55% of which failed to produce positive outcomes because of excessive irradiance delivery, according to guidelines set by the World Association for Laser Therapy. [43] Although randomized, double-blind, placebo-controlled, clinical trials (RCTs) are considered to be the gold standard of scientific research studies, incorrect dosages and setting of the lasers and LEDs used in those studies fully sabotaged any possibility of any positive results within these studies.

There also still remains the controversial questions which remain to be conclusively settled as to whether a coherent monochromatic laser is

---

[43] 2020. [online] Available at: <https://www.ncbi.nlm.nih.gov/pmc/articles/PMC521587 0/> [Accessed 20 May 2020].

superior to non-coherent LEDs typically having a 30 nm band-pass (full width half maximum). Although wavelengths in the NIR region (800–1100 nm) have been the most often used, red wavelengths have sometimes been used either alone, or in combination with NIR. Power levels have also varied markedly from Class IV lasers with total power outputs in the region of 10 W [53], to lasers with more modest power levels (circa 1 W). LEDs can also have widely varying total power levels depending on the size of the array and the number and power of the individual diodes. A low dose of light is beneficial, but raising the dose produces progressively less benefit until eventually a damaging effect can be produced at very high light. It is often said in this context that "more does not mean more," in addition, it should be noted that Class IV lasers are almost too powerful for therapeutic human use, in that is Class IV lasers that start having the dangerous effect of burning human tissue, with the retina of the eyes being the most vulnerable to significant injury. One method for us to know which specific type of PBMT laser or LED is suitable for safe therapeutic healing and cognitive enhancement is to utilize the cumulative data gathered from the successful published scientific trials included in this chapter such as those from Dr. Hamblin's research from Harvard Medical School, which are included in this chapter.

Safety and efficacy studies of PBMT with patients who needed healing from stroke

The first of two studies to test the safety of laser therapy (PMBT) was conducted on 120 stroke patients between the ages of 40 to 85 years of age with a diagnosis of ischemic stroke involving a neurological deficit that could be measured. The purpose of this first clinical trial was to demonstrate the safety and effectiveness of laser therapy for stroke within 24 hours. The researchers in this study found that tPBM significantly improved outcome in human stroke patients, when applied at approximately 18 hours post-stroke, over the entire surface of the head.

The second clinical trial, enrolled 660 patients, aged 40 to 90, who were randomly assigned to one of two groups. Beneficial results were found for moderate and moderate-severe stroke patients. PBM in human subjects who had suffered from severe or even moderate TBI have very long-lasting and even life-changing sequelae (headaches, cognitive impairment, and difficulty sleeping) that prevent them from working or living any kind of normal life. These individuals may have been high achievers before the accident that caused damage to their brains. Initially,

Naeser published a report describing two cases she treated with PBM applied to the forehead twice a week. A 500 mW continuous wave LED source (a mixture of 660 nm red and 830 nm NIR LEDs) with a power density of 22.2 mW/cm^2 (area of 22.48 cm^2), was applied to the forehead for a typical duration of 10 min (13.3 J/cm^2). In the first case study, the patient reported that she could concentrate on tasks for a longer period (the time able to work at a computer increased from 30 min to 3 h). She had a better ability to remember what she read, decreased sensitivity when receiving haircuts in the spots where PBMT was applied, and improved mathematical skills after undergoing PBMT. The second patient had statistically significant improvements compared to prior neuropsychological tests after 9 months of treatment. The patient had a 2 standard deviation (SD) increase on tests of inhibition and inhibition accuracy (9th percentile to 63rd percentile on the Stroop test for executive function and a 1 SD increase on the Wechsler Memory scale test for the logical memory test.

In normal human volunteers, they used transcranial PBM (1064 nm laser, 60 J/cm^2 at 250 mW/cm^2) delivered to the forehead in a placebo-controlled, randomized study, to influence cognitive tasks related to the prefrontal cortex, including a psychomotor vigilance task (PVT), a delayed match-to-sample (DMS) memory task, and the positive and negative affect schedule (PANAS-X) to show improved mood. Subsequent studies in normal humans showed that tPBM with 1064 nm laser could improve performance in the Wisconsin Card Sorting Task (considered the gold standard test for executive function testing). They also showed that tPBM to the right forehead (but not the left forehead) had better effects on improving attention bias modification (ABM) in humans with depression.

Dr. Hamblin also highlighted in an interview with Input magazine that "Many investigators believe that PBM for brain disorders will become one of the most important medical applications of light therapy in the coming years and decades. Despite the efforts of "Big Pharma," prescription drugs for psychiatric disorders are not generally regarded very highly (by both the medical profession nor by the public) because many of these drugs perform little better than placebos in many different trials, and can also have major downside of various negative side-effects."

Laser light therapy, however, has continued to win FDA approval for its healing and regeneration of human tissue capabilities. For example, oral surgeons can now utilize a Laser Assisted New Attachment

Procedure (LANAP) to stimulate oral stem cells, particularly fibroblasts, to form the necessary cellular components that are needed for the patient to organically regenerate healthy tissues in previously diseased root surfaces. The lasers that are used in this procedure have a near-infrared wavelength of 1064 nm that passes through healthy tissue and is selectively absorbed in bacteria and diseased tissues in patient's mouths, all without harming nearby healthy tissues. The energy from this laser can penetrate 4–6 mm beyond the tissue of the mouth's surface to kill bacteria, thereby eliminating infection and inflammation. Once the mouth has been cleared of infectious agents, the laser interacts with hemoglobin to seal the gums with stable fibrin clotting to achieve a clean, closed environment to create regeneration. Multiple peer-reviewed, post-procedure studies tracking results over time show increased regeneration of healthy tissues and continued improvement of oral health using this Laser Assisted Procedure.[44]

PBMT considered as a weapon to fight against our nation's ongoing opioid abuse epidemic. Congress issues a $2.7 million grant to Shepherd University in West Virginia for the study of replacing opioids with PBMT pain control

In 2019, Dr. Kelly Watson Huffer, assistant professor of nursing and IMPACT project manager, said this Congressional grant will allow Shepherd University, which is at the center of our nation's opioid epidemic, to bring innovative therapies and

---

[44] 2020. [online] Available at: <https://www.biooopticsworld.com/biophotonics-tools/article/16430664/fda-approves-laser-procedure-that-stimulates-regrowth-of-oral-tissue-bone> [Accessed 9 May 2020].

treatment modalities such as PBMT and telehealth into Shepherd's curriculum and to the community health centers. "We want to put the additional photobiomodulation (PBMT) equipment out there in the community in the hands of our students and get them to start using it in the clinics," Dr. Huffer says. "Chronic pain is a huge problem all across the country. Certainly, West Virginia has its problems with opioid abuse and overdoses. We're hoping the PBMT technology will help intervene in that."

In a study published in 2006 in the journal *Photomedicine and Laser Surgery*, researchers investigated in a gold standard randomized placebo-controlled trial whether PBMT could benefit humans in acute pain, suffering from soft-tissue injuries. The researchers stated that "there is strong evidence from 19 out of 22 controlled laboratory studies that LLLT can modulate inflammatory pain by reducing levels of biochemical markers. Four comparisons against non-steroidal anti-inflammatory drugs (NSAIDs) in animal studies found optimal doses of LLLT and NSAIDs to be equally effective in the reduction of pain. The researchers concluded in this study that LLLT aka PBMT can modulate inflammatory processes in a dose-dependent manner and can be titrated to significantly reduce acute inflammatory pain in clinical settings. [45]

[45] 2020. [online] Available at: <https://www.liebertpub.com/doi/abs/10.1089/pho.2006.24.158> [Accessed 24 May 2020].

Scientific research finds PBMT to be effective for organically healing within Osteoarthritic Joints. Aching knees and shoulders rejoice!

Another study published in 2009 in the journal *Photomedicine and Laser Surgery* was a gold standard (double-blind randomized placebo-controlled trial) research study investigating whether PBMT could reduce knee pain from osteoarthritis, whether PBMT could increase the microcirculation blood flow within the knee, and whether or not knee flexion could improve. The researchers in this study concluded the experiment by stating in the affirmative that, "In the group treated with active low level laser therapy (LLLT), a significant improvement was found in pain, pressure sensitivity, and flexion. In the placebo group, changes in joint flexion and pain were not significant. Our results show that LLLT reduces pain in knee osteoarthritis (KOA) and improves microcirculation in the irradiated area." [46]

In a study published in 2012, the journal *Ortopedia, Traumatologia, Rehabilitacja* published how researchers investigated the influence of various laser therapy methods on knee joint pain and function in patients with knee osteoarthritis. The scientists in this study concluded that laser irradiation at a dose of 8 J per point and two-wave laser irradiation with doses of 12.4 J and 6.6 J per point significantly

---

[46] 2020. [online] Available at: <https://www.liebertpub.com/doi/abs/10.1089/pho.2008.2297> [Accessed 24 May 2020].

improved knee joint function and relieving knee pain in patients with osteoarthritis. [47]

In a study published in 2016 in the *Journal of Biomedical Optics*, researchers investigated the effectiveness of PBMT in an animal study where the scientists concluded that "The results of this study indicate that PBMT is the most effective therapy in stopping disease progression, and improving inflammatory conditions observed in osteoarthritis." [48] PBMT has had a long proven history of positive effects in the veterinary field.

---

[47] 2020. [online] Available at: <https://europepmc.org/article/med/22764339> [Accessed 24 May 2020].

[48] 2020. [online] Available at: <https://www.spiedigitallibrary.org/journals/Journal-of-Biomedical-Optics/volume-21/issue-10/108001/Isolated-and-combined-effects-of-photobiomodulation-therapy-topical-nonsteroidal-

In a study published in 2016 in the journal *Lasers in Medical Science*, researchers conducted another gold standard research study (double-blind randomized placebo-controlled trial) to investigate the effectiveness of PBMT in skeletal muscle recovery following exercise and concluded that PBMT used as a single treatment is the best modality for enhancement of post-exercise restitution, leading to complete recovery to baseline levels from 24 h after high-intensity eccentric contractions. [49] Weekend warriors and professional athletes are adopting this therapy into their recovery routines as the scientific data and anecdotal positive reviews and testimonitals

anti/10.1117/1.JBO.21.10.108001.full?SSO=1> [Accessed 24 May 2020].

[49] 2020. [online] Available at: <https://link.springer.com/article/10.1007/s10103-016-2071-z> [Accessed 24 May 2020].

significantly increased significantly in the past few years.

In a 2019 study published from the *2019 SBFoton International Optics and Photonics Conference*, researchers evaluated the effects of laser photobiomodulation as a non-pharmacological therapy for pain reduction and improve the quality of life in patients diagnosed with osteoarthritis of the knee. The results, indicating a decrease of the pain and stiffness improvement, demonstrate that BPM is an efficient non-pharmacological therapy for the management of knee osteoarthritis. [50]

In a systematic review study published in 2018 in the journal of *Photomedicine and Laser Surgery,*

---

[50] 2020. [online] Available at: <https://ieeexplore.ieee.org/document/8910257> [Accessed 24 May 2020].

researchers examined six other research studies to evaluate the efficacy of high-intensity laser therapy (PBMT) in the treatment of knee osteoarthritis. The researchers concluded that PBMT seems to be efficient in reducing pain and for providing functional improvements in patients with knee osteoarthritis. [51]

In a study published in 2019 in the journal *Lasers in Medical Science*, scientists investigated the effects of the incorporation of photobiomodulation into a physical exercise program on the level of pain, lower limb muscle strength, and physical capacity, in patients with knee osteoarthritis (OA). Sixty-two female volunteers with a diagnosis of knee OA were distributed into 4 groups for this particular experiment. The scientists concluded this study by

---

[51] 2020. [online] Available at: <https://www.liebertpub.com/doi/abs/10.1089/pho.2017.4425> [Accessed 24 May 2020].

stating that physical exercise and PBMT showed analgesic (pain relieving) effects. [52]

The Spirit of PBMT

In the tapestry of healing, amidst the shadows of pain, a celestial dance of red light unfolds—a symphony of hope, a balm for the soul. Laser red light therapy, like a phoenix rising from the embers, breathes life into the wounded, whispering tales of rejuvenation and grace.

Through the darkness, a crimson beam pierces the veil, tracing delicate patterns upon the canvas of skin. It knows no prejudice, no boundaries, for its love embraces all who seek solace. With gentle caresses, it

---

[52] 2020. [online] Available at: <https://link.springer.com/article/10.1007/s10103-019-02807-3> [Accessed 24 May 2020].

touches the afflicted, igniting a symphony of warmth within.

As the scars of yesterday fade, so do the burdens of the heart. In the tender embrace of red light, pain finds release, and anguish surrenders to peace. Each pulse of radiance carries the promise of a new beginning, of healing unbound by time or space.

In the quiet chambers of the soul, the dance of red light weaves its magic, infusing strength where there was weakness, hope where there was despair. The tears of anguish once shed now glisten with newfound resilience, for the red light's tender touch has transformed sorrow into grace.

Beyond the realm of science, lies the realm of miracles, where red light breathes life into the dormant seeds of faith. Like the embrace of a loving mother, it cradles the weary, guiding them back to the shores of vitality.

Let not the sorrows of yesterday dim the light within, for the laser red light therapy beckons, calling forth the embers of courage and resilience. It whispers, "You are not alone," and in that sacred reassurance, hearts find solace and strength.

So, let the crimson rays wash over you, engulfing you in their tender embrace. Let the rhythm of healing guide your steps, and in the symphony of red light, let your soul be set free. For in the beauty of vulnerability, we find the courage to heal, to transcend, and to rise.

In the tapestry of healing, amidst the shadows of pain, the symphony of red light continues its dance—a testament to the resilience of the human spirit, an ode to the triumph of hope over despair.

Embrace the warmth, embrace the light, for within its gentle glow, lies the key to liberation—an eternal symphony of love and restoration, etched forever in the heart's deepest chambers.

FAQs

In recent years, the field of photobiomodulation, also known as red light laser therapy, has emerged as a groundbreaking approach to promote healing and improve various health conditions.

What is Photobiomodulation?

Photobiomodulation (PBM) is a non-invasive, painless, and drug-free therapeutic technique that utilizes specific wavelengths of light, typically in the red or near-infrared spectrum, to stimulate cellular processes within the body. This light energy penetrates the skin and interacts with cells to trigger various biological responses, leading to healing and tissue repair.

How Does Photobiomodulation Work?

The primary mechanism behind photobiomodulation is the activation of mitochondria within cells. Mitochondria are often referred to as the "powerhouses of the cell" because they play a crucial role in producing energy (ATP) that fuels cellular functions. When exposed to specific wavelengths of light, the activity of mitochondria is enhanced, leading to increased energy production and improved cellular function.

Furthermore, photobiomodulation also promotes the release of nitric oxide, a molecule that helps dilate blood vessels, improves blood flow, and reduces inflammation. These combined effects contribute to tissue repair, reduced pain, and enhanced healing processes.

Applications of Photobiomodulation

Pain Management

Photobiomodulation has shown promising results in alleviating acute and chronic pain conditions. It is commonly used to treat musculoskeletal injuries, arthritis, and neuropathic pain. By reducing inflammation and promoting tissue repair, PBM offers a non-invasive alternative to conventional pain management methods.

Wound Healing

In both acute and chronic wounds, photobiomodulation can accelerate the healing process. By enhancing cell proliferation and tissue regeneration, PBM helps wounds close more rapidly and may reduce the risk of infection.

Skin Rejuvenation

Red light laser therapy is increasingly used in the field of aesthetics for skin rejuvenation. It can stimulate collagen production, improve skin elasticity, and reduce the appearance of fine lines and wrinkles. As a result, photobiomodulation is gaining popularity in the beauty and wellness industry.

Sports Performance and Recovery

Athletes and fitness enthusiasts are incorporating photobiomodulation into their training routines to enhance performance and speed up recovery. By reducing muscle fatigue, inflammation, and promoting tissue repair, PBM can improve athletic performance and reduce the risk of sports-related injuries.

Neurological Disorders

Research is underway to explore the potential of photobiomodulation in managing neurological conditions such as traumatic brain injuries, stroke, and neurodegenerative diseases. While the field is still evolving, early studies have shown promising results.

Hair Regrowth

In cases of androgenetic alopecia (male-pattern baldness) and other hair loss conditions, photobiomodulation has been investigated as a potential treatment to stimulate hair regrowth. By promoting blood flow to hair follicles and increasing cellular activity, PBM may support hair growth.

The Photobiomodulation Process: What to Expect

Photobiomodulation sessions are typically performed by trained professionals using specialized light-emitting devices but are now commonplace and available for purchase by the layperson. The duration and frequency of sessions may vary depending on the condition being treated and the specific device used.

During a photobiomodulation session, the patient will be positioned comfortably, and the light-emitting device will be applied to the targeted area. The red or near-infrared light is then directed onto the skin, and the patient will feel a warm, gentle sensation. The procedure is painless and non-invasive, allowing individuals to resume their daily activities immediately after the session.

Is Photobiomodulation Safe?

Photobiomodulation is considered safe when performed by trained professionals or adults who using appropriate equipment such as eye protective googles, especially with higher power Class 3 and 4 therapeutic lasers. It is a non-ionizing form of light therapy, meaning it does not carry the risks associated with ionizing radiation. However, as with any medical treatment, it is essential to consult with a healthcare professional to determine if photobiomodulation is suitable for individual health conditions and needs.

How long does a typical photobiomodulation session last?

The duration of a photobiomodulation session can vary depending on the condition being treated and the specific device used. Sessions may last anywhere from a few minutes to around 30 minutes.

Are there any side effects of photobiomodulation?

Photobiomodulation is generally considered safe and well-tolerated. However, some individuals may experience mild and temporary effects, such as warmth or redness at the treatment site.

Can photobiomodulation be used alongside other medical treatments?

Yes, photobiomodulation can often be used as an adjunctive therapy alongside other medical treatments. However, it's essential to consult with healthcare professionals to ensure compatibility and safety.

How many photobiomodulation sessions are typically required for hair regrowth?

The number of photobiomodulation sessions needed for hair regrowth can vary depending on individual factors and the severity of the hair loss condition. A series of sessions over several weeks may be recommended for best results.

Is photobiomodulation suitable for children?

Photobiomodulation can be considered for children under appropriate medical supervision. However, individual health conditions and needs should be assessed by healthcare professionals.

Conclusion

Photobiomodulation, or red light laser therapy, is a revolutionary approach to enhance healing, reduce pain, and improve overall well-being. By harnessing the power of specific wavelengths of light, this non-invasive and drug-free therapy offers a range of potential benefits across various medical and aesthetic applications. As research in this field continues to expand, photobiomodulation holds the promise of transforming the way we approach health and wellness.

Chapter 3- Hyperbaric Oxygen Therapy (HBOT) and its neurostimulating plus health recovery benefits.

In previous chapters, we've discussed the technology behind transcranial direct current stimulation, therapeutic lasers and LED lights to stimulate various parts of the body including the brain towards healing, regeneration, and optimal functioning. Now, we'll look at the science and stories behind about how Hyperbaric Oxygen Therapy (HBOT) can add a boost to another critical dimension of brain health and human performance through the ever-important method of increasing blood flow and oxygenation not only throughout our bodies, but especially to every critical region of the brain.

Dr. Daniel Amen is an award-winning psychiatrist, brain-imaging expert, and 10-time New

York Times bestselling author that relies heavily on Hyperbaric Oxygen Therapy (HBOT) in his clinics to "optimize brain health to enable success in all areas of life – relationships, work, finances, passion, and purpose.[53]

One of the main reasons why you will find that Dr. Amen utilizes HBOT to optimize brain and overall health in his clinics is because its a medical technology that has been scientifically proven for decades to be an effective tool for restoring brain health and functioning. HBOT has existed as a FDA-approved treatment for wound healing, carbon monoxide poisoning, burns, and decompression sickness, soft tissue necrosis, and many more indications, but behind those uses, HBOT has also been shown to be

---

[53] 2020. [online] Available at: <https://www.amenclinics.com/about-us/> [Accessed 5 May 2020].

extremely helpful with many other health and human performance issues. HBOT has been shown to help slow the progression of serious memory problems and have a unique capability of improving some traumatic brain injuries, through the mechanism of increasing blood flow to regions of the brain that otherwise would be without adequate blood flow. In addition to sharper recall, some individuals who have utilized HBOT have also reported quicker reaction times in speech, thought, overall cognition, and memory. In addition, HBOT has been found in scientific literature to also be effective for enhancing mitochondrial function, generating new blood vessels, boosting the immune system, increasing stem cell and ATP production, supporting the white blood cells' ability to fight infection, helping the body build new connective tissue, an adjunct for chronic pain therapies, and may even kill certain types of harmful bacteria. [54]

Dr. Daniel Amen frequently uses the story of the NFL Hall of Fame quarterback and living legend Joe Namath, who was having trouble with his cognitive abilities after having competed at the highest levels in the National Football League. Joe experienced an initial 40 sessions of HBOT and was surprised to see that his SPECT functional brain scans started to show remarkable improvements in the blood flow to certain parts of his brain that were not originally receiving adequate blood flow. Joe's SPECT scans had revealed that all of those concussions that he had accumulated on the football field over the years had indeed taken a serious toll on his brain in

---

[54] 2020. [online] Available at: <https://www.amenclinics.com/blog/intensive-healing-for-your-brain/> [Accessed 15 May 2020].

the form of traumatic brain injury (TBI). "With my SPECT scan, I could see the cells on the left side of my head from the forehead back were not getting enough blood flow. Those areas were showing up darker than the rest of the other regions of my brain," Joe says. SPECT brain scans differ from MRI or CT scans. MRI and CT scans are able to show structural damage to the brain but do not reveal how the brain is functioning. In fact, in many people who have suffered a head injury, MRI and CT scans will appear normal even when there is functional damage to the brain. Because SPECT scans are able to reveal any regions of the brain that may not be receiving normal amounts of blood flow, it is often touted as the best tool to use for detecting any functional damage that the brain may have.

Joe Namath went through another 40 sessions of HBOT, and his brain scans showed an even better blood flow to the regions of his brain than before. The dark areas seen on the scans of his brain which had inadequate blood flow had started to lighten up even more and more on subsequent scans and most importantly, he started noticing that his quality of life and health was significantly turning around for the better. After a total of 120 sessions of HBOT, Joe's SPECT scans showed that all of his brain activity was completely restored to normal once again. Since then, Joe was so ecstatic and overjoyed with his improvements that he made it his mission in life from that point forward to spread to the word about the benefits of SPECT brain imaging and hyperbaric oxygen therapy (HBOT) through the Joe Namath Neurological Research Center at Jupiter Medical Center in Florida. "This could help millions," he said, such as "...for the veterans that get concussions, the

children that fall off bicycles and hit their head." [55]
Other NFL players that frequently use hyperbaric
chambers to optimize their recovery from professional
sports wear and tear and injuries include former
Georgia Bulldogs Benjamin Watson and Hines Ward,
Atlanta Falcons QB Matt Schaub, RB Reggie Bush,
Steelers LB James Harrison, and Tim Tebow. Athletes
outside of the NFL that uses regularly use hyperbaric
chambers to enhance their health and performance
include the MLB's Matt Kemp, Rafael Soriano, Adrian
Beltre, UFC star Urijah Faber, Olympic Champion
Michael Phelps, and golf legend Tiger Woods, among
many more.

Dr. Amen and his clinics are particularly
famous around the world for having built the world's

---

[55] 2020. [online] Available at:
<https://www.amenclinics.com/blog/nfl-legend-joe-
namath-says-hyperbaric-oxygen-therapy-healed-his-
damaged-brain/> [Accessed 16 May 2020].

largest database of functional brain scans—over 150,000 and growing. [56] He states that "Brain imaging studies using SPECT show that people who have had HBOT receive marked improvement in blood flow to the brain, which is critical for neuroplasiticity, brain health, and overall health and human performance. SPECT scans are especially unique because they have also been able to reveal how low blood flow is commonly linked to mental health issues, such as ADD/ADHD, depression, bipolar disorder, schizophrenia, addictions, and more." In fact, low blood flow is the #1 brain imaging predictor that an individual will develop Alzheimer's disease, according to Dr. Amen.

---

[56] 2020. [online] Available at: <https://www.amenclinics.com/services/brain-spect/> [Accessed 8 May 2020].

HBOT is a therapy that involves breathing 100% pure oxygen inside of a pressurized chamber, one that is either made from metal such as in the larger unites used in hospitals, or made up of a soft vinyl outer material for those who prefer smaller at-home use. While a person breathes normally inside a HBOT chamber, their lungs take in up to 3 times more oxygen than compared to when they are breathing at normal air pressure because the chamber is pressurized, this helps oxygen to enter your body more easily than at normal atmospheric pressures. The increased oxygen is picked up via the bloodstream and transported all throughout the body and brain, but especially to damaged tissues, facilitating and boosting the body's natural healing process. Although HBOT has some research studies saying that HBOT has no reproducible positive effects for certain patient populations and disease states, more and more recent research and scientific literature are starting to reveal why it is that the off-label use of HBOT within doctors' offices, within professional sports teams, and even inside the homes of many celebrities, biohackers, and athletes are becoming ever more commonplace.

Whenever there is an injury to your body, you need to have an increased amount oxygen to help repair the damaged tissues.[57] Following certain types of injuries, our bodies may demand more oxygen than is available in the normal air we breathe to supply our cells with the fuel necessary for healing processes in metabolism, cellular growth, and repair.[58] Whenever there is a lack of adequate supply of oxygen to any our body's

---

[57] 2020. [online] Available at: <https://www.amenclinics.com/services/hyperbaric-oxygen-therapy/> [Accessed 5 May 2020].
[58] 2020. [online] Available at: <https://www.ncbi.nlm.nih.gov/books/NBK499535/> [Accessed 5 May 2020].

organs, extremities and especially to injured areas, the natural healing mechanisms of our body are not able to work as well as they otherwise could be.

A plethora of new scientific research reveals the effectiveness of HBOT in restoring cognition, providing pain relief, and faster rehabilitation times.

Dr. Amen's clinic website shares the results of a study in 2019 involving SPECT scans that allowed scientists to document improvements in brain metabolism in a patient with Alzheimer's disease. The subject of the study was a 58-year-old woman whose cognitive function had been declining for 5 years. She underwent 40 sessions of HBOT. After just 21 sessions, she reported better mood, a boost in energy, and a better ability to perform routine tasks. She also reported that it was easier for her to do the crossword puzzle. After a total of 40 sessions of HBOT, she reported improvements in concentration, memory, sleep, and ability to use the computer! She also noted a decrease in disorientation, less frustration, and her anxiety was gone as well. Her SPECT brain scans showed a 6.5-38% improvement in overall brain metabolism.[59]

In 2018, the largest published study on HBOT of its kind with a cohort of 154 patients suffering from chronic neurocognitive damage due to traumatic brain injury (TBI), HBOT was associated with significant cognitive improvements. The researchers in this study reported that after treatment with HBOT, there was,

---

[59] 2020. [online] Available at: <https://www.amenclinics.com/services/hyperbaric-oxygen-therapy/> [Accessed 5 May 2020].

"Improvement in memory, improvement of executive functions, and improvement in attention." [60]

In 2019, a gold standard randomized control trial research conducted in Denmark and published in the *Journal of Pain Research* shows that neuroplasticity and pain control were achieved in both short term as well as in the long term after just a single HBOT treatment. The scientists reported that "Our data clearly demonstrated that HBOT has not only acute but also long-lasting neuroplasticity effects on central sensitization." Neuroplasticity in this context means that the body's nervous system was able to improve, adapt, and rehabilitate from its injuries- in other words to bounce back from injury. Neuroplasticity is the ever important function of our

---

[60] 2020. [online] Available at: <https://bmjopen.bmj.com/content/8/9/e023387> [Accessed 5 May 2020].

brains that leads to functional and structural alterations in the nervous system and is intimately linked to not only memory processing, storage, and consolidation, but also enables the modulation of ascending and descending nervous system control pathways, as was observed in this specific study. The researchers concluded that "The present study demonstrates that hyperbaric oxygen therapy has an immediate mitigating effect, as well as a long-lasting preconditioning effect, on secondary hyperalgesia."[61] This is one reason why HBOT has been found to be so useful in its off label use for treating patients with various chronic pain syndromes, such as fibromyalgia.

In February of 2020, hyperbaric oxygen therapy (HBOT) was shown to stimulate improved heart functionality in normal healthy aging

---

[61] https://www.dovepress.com/a-single-session-of-hyperbaric-oxygen-therapy-demonstrates-acute-and-l-peer-reviewed-fulltext-article-JPR

humans, according to a study by the Sagol Center for Hyperbaric Medicine and Research at Shamir Medical Center in Be'er Ya'acov, Israel.

In this research study, the director of the Sagol Center for Hyperbaric Medicine and Research at Shamir Medical Center, Professor Shai Efrati and Dr. Marina Leitman, head of the Echocardiography Unit and Noninvasive Cardiology Service at Shamir Medical Center conducted research with healthy patients who received HBOT to improve cognitive function. These patients underwent a 60-session HBOT treatment course for the study cognitive improvements, but attention was turned HBOT's positive impact on cardiac function as well, when they noticed that 31 patients who were evaluated using a high-resolution echocardiography had amazingly been identified as having had the remarkable effect of generation of new blood vessels (angiogenesis) and tissue regeneration around their hearts!

HBOT's ability to improve mitochondrial function may explain the beneficial effects that we saw in the cardiac function of this normal aging population said Dr. Leitman. In recent years, there is growing evidence on the regenerative effects of HBOT. We have now realized that the combined action of both hyperoxia (an excess of oxygen in the body) and hyperbaric pressure together, leads to significant improvement in tissue oxygenation while targeting both oxygen and pressure-sensitive genes, resulting in improved mitochondrial metabolism with anti-apoptotic (anti-cell death) and anti-inflammatory effects," according to Dr. Efrati.

The newly developed protocols used in this study, which included the intermittent increasing and decreasing oxygen concentration, were especially capable for stimulating within the body what is known as the "Hyperoxic – Hypoxic Paradox." This, he says "induces stem cell proliferation and mobilization, leading to the generation of new blood vessels, called angiogenesis, and tissue regeneration."

Dr. Efrati said that during the first studies they conducted at the Sagol Center, they had evaluated the beneficial effects of HBOT in treating traumatic brain injury and stroke. "However, in this study, we evaluated for the very first time the effect of new HBOT protocols on the "normal" aging heart. For the first time in humans, we have demonstrated that HBOT can improve cardiac function as well."
Efrati said for the last 12 years his team has developed an ongoing research program "that investigates the regenerative effects of HBOT on different issues and on different degrees of damage to human tissues. The researchers found that HBOT induced many of the essential elements crucial to repairing almost any mechanism within the human body.

Along with normal aging, there is typically a marked decrease in cardiac function – particularly in the mitochondrial cells of the heart, Efrati said. "Mitochondria cells are the 'powerhouse" cells of the body and this is where we create energy," he said. "HBOT's ability to improve mitochondrial function may explain the beneficial effects that we saw in the cardiac function of this normal aging population."

By exposing the mitochondria to the fluctuations in oxygen by the use of HBOT, the team observed "an improvement in contractility function of the heart – meaning, the heart muscle also contracted much more efficiently over the course of a 60-session HBOT protocol."

Dr. Efrati also noted that the effect was particularly evident in the left ventricle, which is the chamber responsible for pumping oxygenated blood to the rest of the body. This is only the beginning of our understanding of the impact of HBOT on cardiac function in a normally aging population, and a larger and more diverse cohort will be required to further evaluate our initial findings, he said. Asked whether this treatment could also be used on people who are predisposed to heart conditions, Efrati said the short answer is "yes," but he stressed that more research is needed. "As far as we know, we are the first to identify HBOT's ability to improve cardiac function. Our study was on a group of 31 asymptomatic normal aging heart patients."[62]

Dr. Salerno is a famous functional medicine doctor with a clinical practice in New York City that is a popular destination for numerous celebrities and

---

[62] 2020. [online] Available at: <https://www.jpost.com/health-science/hyperbaric-oxygen-therapy-improves-heart-function-in-healthy-aging-people-616391> [Accessed 5 May 2020].

famous athletes. In an interview, he says that he was actually prompted to get a HBOT chamber at his medical clinic at the personal request of self-help guru Tony Robbins. Tony, is one of many celebrities and athletes who swear upon the use of Hyperbaric Oxygen Therapy as one of their most preferred adjuncts for health and human performance.

Dr. Salerno explains how hyperbaric chambers can bolster the body's own natural healing process

"With the additional oxygen going into your bloodstream with HBOT, you are delivering the most basic and valuable nutrients that your tissue needs to survive and thrive. When the inflammation is pushed out, and the tissue is revived from fresh blood delivery through the vascular system, the healing process improves, a lessened inflammatory response is seen in patients with autoimmunity conditions like multiple sclerosis or rheumatoid arthritis, and shortened recovery times are reported by professional athletes in the NFL. Increased rate of recovery times while using the chamber is what many athletes utilize HBOT for, but many also report anecdotally that HBOT seems to also generate glowing skin and improve skin elasticity, improved brain function, memory, and mood" says Dr. Salerno. [63]

---

[63] 2020. [online] Available at: <https://www.huffpost.com/entry/8-life-changing-benefits_b_13682436?guccounter=1&guce_referrer=aHR0cHM6Ly93d3cuZ29vZ2xlLmNvbS8&guce_referrer_sig=AQAAAF2RPL4bD-XXg_VRJATuBovP_UuUhDjln0VwkNmIwt67nsUQpWL5ntk2Uug9rAgm-z22TDGlxNzqXoeHDUlbKOtg4QO2BBCNcB8gdgc7TpEN_gEZHHk8_d0W7w6ghh4U9ssNkah01NUWcD08iXEf9Ju5AjP4aFbpfhtslzFq3yCf> [Accessed 5 May 2020].

In a USA today news interview, Steve Weatherford of the New York Giants, stated that many of his fellow NFL players personally own HBOT chambers in their homes. "Despite how futuristic sleeping in hyperbaric chamber may seem, this has actually become a common practice among many NFL players for a few years now. I have my own portable chamber in my house. The reason why I and so many NFL players sleep in these chambers is because a hyperbaric chamber reduces swelling, promotes the healing of wounds, helps fight off dangerous infections, and increases the amount of oxygen in the bloodstream. [64]

Ben Greenfield is just one of many such top-ranked athletes and biohackers who utilize HBOT

[64] 2020. [online] Available at: <https://ftw.usatoday.com/2015/12/steve-weatherford-explains-why-nfl-players-often-sleep-in-hyperbaric-chambers> [Accessed 8 May 2020].

regularly to optimize personal health, wellness, and athletic performance. In 2013 and 2014, Ben was named as one of the world's top 100 most influential people in health and fitness. In 2016, he joined Spartan SGX as one of its certified coaches. Ben most notably won the Gold Medal for the USA in a long course triathlon race in the ITU world triathlon series in 2011 and continues to compete as one of the top-ranked amateur triathletes in the world, completing over 120 races and 12 Ironman triathlons while racing for the elite Team Timex multisport team. He frequently raves about how useful HBOT and infrared sauna within his home is for supercharging his recovery and boosting his athletic performance.

Ben Greenfield stated that perhaps it is because oxygen is an invisible gas and that surrounded by and that breathing is so automatic of a process, that we often just plain forget to think about oxygen as a crucial nutrient for our bodies, our overall health, and crucial to our ability to perform at high levels. But oxygen is a fundamental and absolutely critical component that our body uses for the production of cellular energy (ATP) he says. Ben also goes on to say that many professional athletes have long understood the role oxygen plays in their athletic performance and successes. "This is why athletes train at altitude or take drastic steps like blood doping or using EPO or even free-diving to improve upon their athletic performance. Having more oxygen available to working tissues will improve the tissue's capacity for work. While we are not talking about dramatic increases in oxygen, it is definitely enough to see some performance changes and at the elite athlete level, many will do whatever it takes even to shave a few seconds off their time or gain one extra repetition. There are times that red blood cells might be fully saturated with oxygen, but due to trauma to the circulation system, the human body cannot deliver the oxygen to where it needs to go. This trauma can be macro trauma from an accident or injury and/or microcirculation damage from a long list of things including chronic inflammation, toxicity, overuse injuries, and exercise." [65]

New research studies show the many benefits of HBOT

In 2015, there was a research study of 209 participants, conducted by the Department of Anaesthesia, Prince of Wales Clinical School, University of NSW in Sydney Australia that concluded

---

[65] 2020. [online] Available at: <https://bengreenfieldfitness.com/article/recovery-articles/hyperbaric-oxygen-therapy-benefits/> [Accessed 5 May 2020].

that there was some evidence that HBOT was effective for the termination of acute migraines. [66]

In a 2017 study published in the journal *Undersea & Hyperbaric Medicine*, the researchers concluded that HBOT treatment correlated with stem cell mobilization as well as increased cognitive performance. [67]

In a 2019 study published in the scientific journal *Hyperbaric Oxygen Therapy*, the researchers concluded that after they had treated more than 720 patients suffering from osteomyelitis (infection of the

---

[66] 2020. [online] Available at: <https://www.ncbi.nlm.nih.gov/pubmed/26709672> [Accessed 15 May 2020].
[67] 2020. [online] Available at: <https://europepmc.org/article/med/28779582> [Accessed 24 May 2020].

bone) using HBOT, that it had contributed to the improvement of the patients' treatment results. [68]

The *Journal of Restorative Neurology and Neuroscience* concluded that after having had treated 162 stroke patient with HBOT, significant improvements in all cognitive domains were demonstrated, even in the late chronic stages of the disease. [69]

In a study published in 2020 in the journal *Spine*, the researchers reported that the application of HBOT contributed to the immediate and sustained improvement in motor recovery after

---

[68] 2020. [online] Available at: <https://link.springer.com/chapter/10.1007/978-981-13-7836-2_5> [Accessed 24 May 2020].
[69] 2020. [online] Available at: <https://content.iospress.com/articles/restorative-neurology-and-neuroscience/rnn190959> [Accessed 24 May 2020].

postoperative spinal cord injury. HBOT may represent a new avenue of therapy for spinal cord injury. [70]

In 2011 independent researchers hired by the Department of Veterans Affairs in Washington D.C. stated that HBOT is one innovative treatment being explored for difficult-to-treat conditions, given its remarkable and unique potential to promote healing of the microscopic and macroscopic wounds to the white matter of the brain that have been attributed to traumatic brain injury (TBI) and post-traumatic stress disorder. The scientists recognized that in TBI patients, HBOT improved cerebral blood flow and glucose metabolism. They added that Gene Array Analysis (genetic testing) had also demonstrated positive impacts on gene expression as well.

---

[70] 2020. [online] Available at: <https://journals.lww.com/spinejournal/Abstract/9000/T he_Treatment_of_Perioperative_Spinal_Cord_Injury.9426 3.aspx> [Accessed 24 May 2020].

Controversy still exists within the scientific community regarding the reproducibility of beneficial effects that HBOT is being anecdotally used for. The safety profile of HBOT, however, remains rock solid

There still exists controversy in scientific and academic literature today in regards to the reproducibility of beneficial effects for all of the patient populations and conditions that some studies shown HBOT to be beneficial for. The safety profile of HBOT however is indisputable, undeniable, and continues to speak for itself across all the major scientific publications. Minor ear problems, such as ear pain and barotrauma, appear to be the most common adverse effects of HBOT. HBOT is believed to be generally safe when used as directed for FDA-cleared indications. Per the Undersea and Hyperbaric Medical Society, middle ear barotrauma and sinus squeeze are the 2 most common side effects of hyperbaric oxygen in populations, with an incidence of approximately 2%, which should be noted is exceeding rare. The independent research study of HBOT by the Department of Veterans Affairs above had at least proven useful in stating that there are no clear red flags for serious harms with the use of HBOT as a medical treatment. [71]

In 2017, a significantly massive sized safety study reviewing the usage of 1.5 million HBOT treatments between 2012-2015 was published in the journal *Advances in Skin & Wound Care*. The

---

[71] 2020. [online] Available at: <https://www.ncbi.nlm.nih.gov/books/NBK499535/> [Accessed 5 May 2020].

researchers in this research study also concluded that the occurrence of adverse events over the course of 1.5 million treatments associated with HBO therapy is infrequent and typically not serious. The findings of this study suggest that when administered according to the appropriate therapeutic protocols HBO therapy is a safe and low-risk intervention. [72] As of the time of the writing of this book, the Department of Veterans Affairs still has chosen not to incorporate HBOT as a treatment in all of their veteran's hospitals nationwide, due to their inability to successfully reproduce the positive effects of HBOT for all conditions that it has anecdotally been found useful for, unfortunately. The grassroots demand from Veterans and Veterans' groups have remained high,

[72] 2020. [online] Available at: <https://journals.lww.com/aswcjournal/Abstract/2017/03000/A_Retrospective_Analysis_of_Adverse_Events_in.7.aspx> [Accessed 24 May 2020].

and there are a select few VA hospitals in the country that have started to incorporate HBOT treatments for veterans, in response to their constituent demand.

The Spirit of HBOT

Amidst the depths of healing's embrace, where shadows of affliction fade, there blooms a wondrous tapestry of hope—a dance of hyperbaric oxygen therapy, a symphony of life's renewal.

Beneath the surface of the soul's sanctuary, a chamber of wonder awaits—a sanctuary where oxygen's gentle touch awakens the dormant spirit. Like a tender breeze whispering through ancient forests, the therapy breathes life into every cell, infusing them with the elixir of vitality.

In the belly of the chamber, time dissolves, and the world outside fades away. Here, the heart's rhythm aligns with the cadence of the universe, and the soul finds solace in the ethereal embrace.

Within the depths of darkness, where wounds once lay bare, a gentle glow of hope begins to radiate. With each inhalation, the spirit rises, transcending the shackles of pain, and the symphony of healing resonates through the body's sacred temples.

As the oxygen weaves its magic, the scars of yesterday fade like ink upon parchment, and the spirit finds renewal in the arms of grace. In this ethereal dance, even the most tender wounds find solace, for the therapy's caress knows no boundaries.

The heartbeat of hope echoes in every chamber, a reminder that within us lies the resilience to endure, to transcend, and to heal. Oh, how the oxygen whispers tales of triumph, painting the canvas of the soul with hues of restoration.

Through the hallowed embrace of hyperbaric oxygen therapy, the spirit becomes a phoenix rising from ashes—the embodiment of revival and rebirth. It is a symphony of courage and resilience, a testament to the indomitable human spirit.

So, embrace the therapy's tender touch, for within its ethereal grasp lies the key to liberation. Let it guide you through the labyrinth of healing, illuminating the path to renewal and restoration.

In the depths of healing's embrace, where shadows of affliction once prevailed, there blooms a wondrous tapestry of hope—a dance of hyperbaric oxygen therapy, a symphony of life's renewal.

FAQs

What is Hyperbaric Oxygen Therapy (HBOT)?

Hyperbaric Oxygen Therapy (HBOT) is a non-invasive medical treatment that involves breathing pure oxygen in a pressurized environment. Patients are placed inside a hyperbaric chamber, where the atmospheric pressure is higher than normal, allowing the lungs to take in a higher concentration of oxygen than they would under normal conditions. At home versions of HBOT chambers are often soft-outer shell models, which makes the therapy slightly less effective.

How Does Hyperbaric Oxygen Therapy Work?

During an HBOT session, the increased pressure causes oxygen to dissolve more efficiently in the bloodstream. This oxygen-rich blood is then delivered to tissues and organs throughout the body, even to areas with restricted blood flow or damaged tissues. The heightened oxygen levels promote healing and can enhance the body's natural restorative processes.

Medical Applications of Hyperbaric Oxygen Therapy

Wound Healing

HBOT is widely used for wound healing, especially in cases of chronic non-healing wounds, diabetic ulcers, and radiation-induced tissue damage. The increased oxygen supply accelerates tissue repair and stimulates the growth of new blood vessels.

Carbon Monoxide Poisoning

Hyperbaric Oxygen Therapy is a critical treatment for carbon monoxide poisoning. Breathing pure oxygen at high pressure helps to rapidly clear carbon monoxide from the bloodstream, preventing further damage.

Decompression Sickness

Also known as "the bends," decompression sickness can affect divers who ascend too quickly. HBOT is a standard treatment for this condition, as it reduces the bubbles of gas in the blood and tissues, relieving symptoms and preventing complications.

Radiation Injury

Cancer patients who undergo radiation therapy may experience tissue damage in the treated area. Hyperbaric Oxygen Therapy can aid in the healing of these damaged tissues, improving the quality of life for cancer survivors.

Infections

HBOT can be used as an adjunctive therapy for certain infections, particularly those caused by anaerobic bacteria that thrive in low-oxygen environments. The increased oxygen levels help the body's immune system fight off infections more effectively.

Traumatic Brain Injury (TBI) and Stroke

Research suggests that Hyperbaric Oxygen Therapy may have potential benefits for patients with traumatic brain injuries and stroke. By increasing oxygen delivery to the brain, HBOT may promote healing and reduce inflammation.

The HBOT Procedure: What to Expect

Before beginning an HBOT session, a patient will be briefed about the procedure and any safety precautions. They will then be asked to wear comfortable clothing and remove any items that may pose a fire hazard inside the hyperbaric chamber.

Once inside the chamber, the patient will lie down, and the chamber will be sealed. The pressure inside the chamber will gradually increase, simulating the experience of descending underwater. Patients may experience a sensation of pressure in their ears, similar to what one feels during a flight or scuba diving.

Throughout the session, patients can communicate with the chamber operator via an intercom system.

They are also free to bring books, music, or other forms of entertainment to pass the time during the treatment, which typically lasts for about 60 to 120 minutes.

After the session is complete, the pressure inside the chamber will slowly return to normal, and the patient can safely exit.

Is Hyperbaric Oxygen Therapy Safe?

Hyperbaric Oxygen Therapy is generally considered safe when administered by trained professionals. However, like any medical treatment, there are potential risks and side effects. Some individuals may experience ear discomfort, sinus pain, or changes in vision. It's crucial for patients to disclose any pre-existing medical conditions to their healthcare providers before starting HBOT.

How many HBOT sessions are typically required for wound healing?

The number of HBOT sessions needed for wound healing can vary depending on the individual and the severity of the wound or condition. It is typically recommended to undergo a series of sessions to achieve the best results.

Are there any side effects of Hyperbaric Oxygen Therapy?

While HBOT is generally safe, some individuals may experience mild side effects such as ear discomfort, sinus pain, or changes in vision. These effects are usually temporary and subside after the session.

Can HBOT help with neurological conditions like multiple sclerosis?

There is ongoing research on the potential benefits of HBOT for neurological conditions like multiple sclerosis. While some studies show promising results, more research is needed to establish its effectiveness conclusively.

Is HBOT covered by health insurance?

In some cases, Hyperbaric Oxygen Therapy may be covered by health insurance, especially for approved medical indications. Patients are advised to check with their insurance provider for specific coverage details.

Can children undergo Hyperbaric Oxygen Therapy?

Yes, children can undergo HBOT. However, the decision should be made in consultation with their healthcare provider to ensure it is appropriate for their condition.

Conclusion

Hyperbaric Oxygen Therapy (HBOT) is a fascinating medical treatment that shows promise in various applications. Frequently used by the professional athletic community with a long history of positive reviews, it has become a staple within the biohacker community as well. From wound healing to treating carbon monoxide poisoning to maximizing health and functioning, the increased oxygen levels provided during an HBOT session can have significant therapeutic effects. As research in this field continues, we can expect to see even more potential benefits and applications of Hyperbaric Oxygen Therapy in the future.

Chapter 4- Transcranial magnetic stimulation

"A Life-Saver and a Game-changer." TMS provides a much-needed new treatment option for sufferers

Transcranial Magnetic Stimulation (TMS) is a relatively new brain stimulation technology that is becoming increasingly available in some doctors' offices and also quickly gaining a following of happy satisfied customers. It is a neurostimulation medical device that's currently approved by the Food and Drug Administration (FDA) for the treatment major depression, obsessive-compulsive disorder (OCD), and migraines. TMS functions through copper magnetic coils and a magnetic field, that when hovered over certain portions of the brain, can create a unique form of neuroplasticity and increased blood flow for those who seek improvements for their cognitive health related conditions.

According to a published literature review by Antonio H. Iglesias, MD, a Loyola Medicine neurologist and assistant professor at the Loyola University Chicago Stritch School of Medicine, TMS has shown "significant efficacy in treating major depressive and obsessive-compulsive disorders. TMS has now also opened up the field of neurology in general in multiple areas. Dr. Iglesias says there are currently 1,641 studies underway utilizing TMS to treat a broad array of neurological disorders, including more than 60 trials alone studying the effects of TMS' ability to diminish or reverse the effects of early dementia. The most promising results he says, however, are in the treatment of acute migraines, in primary progressive aphasia, and with the effects of stroke. Unlike transcranial direct current stimulation (tDCS) which uses a small amount of electric current to directly stimulate the brain, TMS is a device that is made of one or two copper coils, positioned over and hovered over a targeted area of a patient's head for a short period of time. The TMS device produces brief magnetic pulses that penetrate the patient's skull to an estimated depth of approximately 2 to 2.5 centimeters. The magnetic field then triggers changes in neuronal activity and communication, which serves to alter unwanted activities within the brain. "TMS can work as a stimulant or an inhibitor of cerebral activity, or both. Most importantly, TMS is well-tolerated by most patients with few side effects," says Dr. Iglesias. [73]

[73] 2020. [online] Available at: <https://scienmag.com/tms-shows-promise-in-treating-stroke-dementia-and-migraines/> [Accessed 3 May 2020].

For migraine sufferers, there are no currently no cures available, according to Dr. Starling, a neurologist at Mayo Clinic, however, "TMS may be a new effective, well-tolerated treatment option for migraine prevention. Migraines are a neurologic disease that can be so incapacitating for people, that it is important to have a variety of new treatment options" to address it. Dr. Amaal Starling is a neurologist at Mayo Clinic and the lead author of a new study that looked at single-pulse transcranial magnetic stimulation for the preventive treatment of migraine, the sixth most disabling neurologic disease globally, a disease that is debilitating for more than 38 million Americans. [74]

---

[74] 2020. [online] Available at: <https://newsnetwork.mayoclinic.org/discussion/mayo-clinic-minute-new-device-can-prevent-migraine-attacks/> [Accessed 3 May 2020].

News articles from both within the USA and worldwide report that many patients who have experienced TMS treatment claim it is "life-saver" and a "game-changer" for their depressive disorders

According to Dr. Adam Stern of Harvard Medical School's Harvard Health Publishing, depression is the leading cause of disability in the United States among people ages 15 to 44. Dr. Stern stated that, "People with depression who have tried and failed to receive benefit from medications can now experience a clinically meaningful response with TMS. About one-third of these individuals who undergo TMS treatments experience a full remission, meaning that their symptoms go away completely", [75] which is incredible and remarkable compared to other types of treatments in the past.

Marcia Terry was a sufferer who had been treated with multiple medications and therapies for her major depressive disorder over the course of many years earlier in her life. Marcia relayed her life story to CBS News in a 2019 interview, exclaiming that she had suffered so immensely from her illness and for almost all of her entire life, to she was at the point where she was so debilitated that she couldn't even leave her home for months at a time. Marcia Terry reported that after having experienced TMS treatment for her disorder, for the first time in her life she has been able to say, "I love life," and "I have so

[75] 2020. [online] Available at: <https://www.health.harvard.edu/blog/transcranial-magnetic-stimulation-for-depression-2018022313335> [Accessed 13 May 2020].

much hope", [76] marking an incredibly profound change in her life's direction and in her outlook in life.

Dr. Marcus DeCarvalho is a psychiatrist from Jacksonville Florida who had treated one of his patients named Gina (she didn't use her real name in this news article due to the stigma attached to having major depression) with TMS therapy. Gina had tried a large number of different medications, counseling, various therapies, self-help books, and more, but none of those modalities had helped her. Depression had robbed her of so much of her normal abilities to function that it had even hospitalized her several times throughout her life. She suffered constantly and for many years because she couldn't eat, sleep, and life became so painful for her that she even admitted

---

[76] 2020. [online] Available at:
<https://www.cbsnews.com/news/deep-transcranial-magnetic-stimulation-changed-womans-life-depression/>
[Accessed 3 May 2020].

that she had tried to take her own life on several occasions. Unless you've experienced major depression, she said, you can't imagine what it feels like. She described her symptoms as "unbearable physical pain," and in her desperate last-ditch effort to ease her depression, Gina decided to try TMS therapy with Dr. DeCarvalho. She exclaimed that for the first time in her life following TMS treatment, she feels like she's on track to actually get better in her life for the first time in a long time and that "TMS had saved her life". [77]

In a similar news article by an overseas affiliate of CBS news in Australia reported on the story of Kate O'Farrell, who was diagnosed with major depression at age 16. The condition forced her in and out of the

---

[77] 2020. [online] Available at: <htttps://www.news4jax.com/health/2018/06/13/non-invasive-depression-treatment-saves-jacksonville-moms-life/> [Accessed 13 May 2020].

hospital, making work or study almost impossible. Like 40 percent of people with serious cases of depression, medication alone didn't work for her. However, after Ms. O'Farrell had tried transcranial magnetic stimulation (TMS), the results were clear, "TMS has been a game-changer for me," she said. 34-year-old Australian actress Anna Kidd Similar had also stated in an Australian ABC news report that, "This is the longest period in my life where I've felt healthy. It (TMS) changed my life." [78]

Stanford University's School of Medicine Dr. Nolan Williams has also been studying the many applications of transcranial magnetic stimulation (TMS) for a wide variety of neurological conditions. In April 2020, a publication from Stanford University

---

[78] 2020. [online] Available at: <https://www.abc.net.au/news/2018-10-11/magnetic-depression-treatment-turning-lives-around/10337174> [Accessed 3 May 2020].

stated that transcranial magnetic brain stimulation treatment had rapidly relieved symptoms of severe depression in an incredible 90% of the study's participants! The treatment protocol is called Stanford Accelerated Intelligent Neuromodulation Therapy, or SAINT for short. The SAINT researchers reported also that they were able to improve upon current FDA-approved protocols by increasing the number of magnetic pulses, speeding up the pace of the treatment, and targeting the pulses according to each individual's neurocircuitry to achieve improvements in TMS therapy, to achieve their incredible results.

The leading world expert on TMS explains how normal healthy brain functioning is restored in TMS treatments

Dr. Nolan Williams is a double board-certified physician and a leading world expert in regards to TMS brain stimulation. He explains, that in the case of depression, it is the left dorsolateral prefrontal cortex, in at least some people, that is hypofunctional, or has decreased functionality in that region. In a simplistic view, he says – all you would need to do is get the magnetic coil over this region and excite it. TMS is an electromagnetic device that produces depolarization of cortical neurons. Primarily what we are doing is that we are inducing an electrical current with a magnetic field – enabling us to pass through low conductive substances and get it only into the brain in precise areas that need help.

There are certain aspects of TMS that certainly seem to mimic psychiatric drugs, except with far more superior results. For instance, the dopamine release that happens after TMS stimulation of the brain's prefrontal cortex is not the same exact thing as having a drug block the reuptake of dopamine, because TMS is instead restoring normal neurophysiological function. In the case of TMS, the beauty is that it's an entirely different approach of trying to change brain network function back to something more physiologically normal, without any pain nor any of the serious negative side effects of pharmaceutical treatments. "The interesting thing is," Dr. Nolan said, "that in the over 500 patients I have treated over the last decade of my life, I have never had a patient come to say, "I feel normal again" those patients that had been treated with psychiatric medications), instead they'll usually say something more like, 'My depression may be gone, but I feel this weird unexplainable side effect."

In a study from 2019, two psychiatrists from the University of Texas at Rio Grande Valley looked at the positive benefit of TMS and reported, "Studies have suggested a correlation between cerebral metabolic activity and TMS effectiveness. This was validated by the results of TMS treatment in previous treatment nonresponders who exhibited hypo-perfusion (low blood flow) in the frontal cortex of their brains. A pilot study that they looked at involving 15 medication-resistant patients demonstrated an increase in cerebral blood volume during TMS. Repeated stimulation also demonstrated increased synaptic plasticity (Neuroplasticity) they stated. They concluded their research paper by stating that TMS is an effective and treatment with few side effects compared to anti-depressant medications." [79]

In another published study in 2019 that was published in the journal <u>Clinical Psychopharmacology and Neuroscience,</u> experimented with 259 patients using TMS. The researchers found that the patients who responded well to TMS, usually have a hyperactive hypothalamic-pituitary-adrenal axis, hence serum cortisol level may predict the relapse of depressive episodes in TMS responders. Similarly, the thyroid function test (free T3, free T4, and thyroid-stimulating hormone (TSH) was evaluated in patients with depression receiving TMS. There was no difference in the pre to post intervention-free T3 and

---

[79] 2020. [online] Available at: <https://search.proquest.com/openview/eec02fecfebc846a0c180d878dd35266/1?pq-origsite=gscholar&cbl=2045583> [Accessed 22 May 2020].

free T4 levels; however, the TSH hormone level was found to be high in TMS responders. [80]

Essential elements of safety in TMS treatments

There are three essential elements to TMS treatments. There is the diagnosis, the target, and the direction of the stimulation. You want to have a diagnosis, what neuroanatomy you are targeting, and which direction to send the brain into. In some cases, if you send the brain in the wrong direction at the right target, you can make symptoms worse. If you stimulate or inhibit the brain at the right target, for the right diagnosis, it is either going to work completely, partially, or not at all. Some physicians

[80] 2020. [online] Available at: <https://www.ncbi.nlm.nih.gov/pmc/articles/PMC6361049/> [Accessed 22 May 2020].

have used TMS to inhibit certain areas that are hyperactive in people with drug-seeking or addictive behaviors. Others have tried to excite areas that are under-active in cases of major depression. You can make the brain fire in a way that makes it more likely to be excitable, or you can send an inhibitory pulse sequence and you can make the brain less likely to be excitable. I have both a clinical TMS practice and a lab in which I run experimental TMS protocols for various problems Dr. Nolan Williams stated. Generally, between those two populations of patients, studying TMS is extraordinarily both rewarding and effective. For an intervention as low risk as this is, something that has only a 1 in 30,000 risks of a short seizure and has never resulted in any long-term problem. I had one lady who was getting treated and was doing fairly well early on treatment, but we found out she was still drinking alcohol, which is a risk for having TMS-related seizures with certain stimulation protocols.

We switched her to one that was not risky from a TMS seizure standpoint. Not only did she have improvement with her depression, but she also stopped drinking, went to AA for the first time in her life, and went back to work. We have seen several people who have had that kind of success. I have another patient with pretty severe OCD, and after a couple of days of treatment was able to leave the hospital and do quite well in the world. To test safety, the researchers evaluated the participants' cognitive function before and after treatment. They found no negative side effects; in fact, they discovered that the participants' ability to switch between mental tasks and to solve problems had improved — a typical outcome for people who are no longer depressed. TMS is not a permanent solution, unfortunately. It is similar to dialysis; in that you have to have treatments with it repeatedly. The good news about TMS, unlike dialysis, is that you can do a six-week course and without any other treatment, about 2/3 of people will maintain a response up to the six-month mark. If you give booster TMS courses, you get it closer to 90% of people maintaining their response. Whether it is a treatment-resistant depression or treatment-resistant OCD, those folks are not at all bothered by this idea of coming back in, they are just happy that they are feeling better. Patients have regularly reported that TMS is a life-changing intervention for them, putting them back on the path of having a normal life, according to Dr. Williams.

When Deirdre Lehman, 60, woke up the morning in 2018, she said she was hit by what she described as "a tsunami of darkness." Lehman had struggled with bipolar disorder all her adult life, but with medications and psychotherapy, her mood had been stable for 15 years.

"There was a constant chattering in my brain: It was my own voice talking about depression, agony, hopelessness," she said. "I told my husband, 'I'm going down and I'm heading toward suicide.' There seemed to be no other option. "Lehman's psychiatrist had heard of the SAINT study and referred her to Stanford. After researchers pinpointed the spot in her brain that would benefit from stimulation, Lehman underwent the therapy.

"By the third round, the chatter started to ease," she said. "By lunch, I could look my husband in the eye. With each session, the chatter got less and less until it was completely quiet. "That was the most peace there's been in my brain since I was 16 and started down the path to bipolar disorder." Since undergoing SAINT treatment, she has completed a bachelor's degree at the University of California-Santa Barbara; she had dropped out as a young woman when her bipolar symptoms overwhelmed her studies.

"I used to cry over the slightest thing," she said. "But when bad things happen now, I'm now just resilient and stable. I'm in a much more peaceful state of mind, able to enjoy the positive things in life with the energy to get things done." Stanford researchers hypothesized that some modifications to transcranial magnetic stimulation could improve its effectiveness. Studies had suggested that a stronger dose, of 1,800 pulses per session instead of 600, would be more effective. The researchers were cautiously optimistic about the safety of the treatment, as that dose of stimulation had been used without harm in other forms of brain stimulation for neurological disorders, such as Parkinson's disease. Other studies suggested that accelerating the treatment would help relieve patients' depression more rapidly. With SAINT, study participants underwent 10 sessions per day of 10-minute treatments, with 50-minute breaks in between. After a day of therapy, Lehman's mood score indicated she was no longer depressed; it took up to five days for other participants. On average, three days of the therapy were enough for participants to have relief from depression. [81]

---

[81] 2020. [online] Available at: <http://med.stanford.edu/news/all-news/2020/04/stanford-researchers-devise-treatment-that-relieved-depression-i.html> [Accessed 3 May 2020].

TMS elicits neuroplasticity, helping those who are interested in achieving optimal brain functioning. Revisiting Harvard Medical School's recommendations for brain health optimization

In 2019, researchers published the results of an experiment called "High-Frequency Repetitive Transcranial Magnetic Stimulation Could Improve Impaired Working Memory Induced by Sleep Deprivation." In the study's conclusion, in regards to the impairment of working memory induced by chronic sleep deprivation, it was stated that it could very well be rescued by repetitive TMS. The improvement of behavioral performance in the sleep-deprived may be attributed to the positive modulation of TMS on the spontaneous neural activity of cognition-related brain areas. Neuronal physiology that responds to TMS is of central importance, as repetitive stimulations increase synaptic plasticity (neuroplasticity), causing it to last longer even after stimulation ceases. [82]

Revisiting Harvard Medical School's website article regarding brain health that was published on January 29, 2020, we can see that the recommendations to keep the brain young and healthy can be uniquely achieved by the TMS modality for those who are driven in the pursuit of becoming the best versions of themselves:

1. Mental stimulation-

Develop more neurological "plasticity" and build up a functional reserve that provides a hedge

---

[82] 2020. [online] Available at: <https://www.hindawi.com/journals/np/2019/7030286/> [Accessed 22 May 2020].

against future cell loss. Any mentally stimulating activity should help to build up your brain.

2. Get physical exercise-

Bring more oxygen-rich blood to the region of the brain that is responsible for thought. Exercise also spurs the development of new nerve cells and increases the connections between brain cells (*synapses*). This results in brains that are more efficient, plastic, and adaptive, which translates into better performance.[83]

---

[83] 2020. [online] Available at: <https://www.health.harvard.edu/mind-and-mood/12-ways-to-keep-your-brain-young> [Accessed 4 May 2020].

Stanford researchers find that TMS strengthens certain weak connections within the brain, while simultaneously calming overactive regions, and enhances overall cognitive functioning

Back at SAINT, the Stanford Medical School researchers use magnetic resonance imaging (MRI) of brain activity to locate not only the dorsolateral prefrontal cortex but a particular sub-region within it. They are able to really pinpoint the areas of the subgenual cingulate, a part of the brain that is overactive in people experiencing depression.

"In people who are depressed, the connection between the dorsolateral prefrontal cortex and the subgenual cingulate is weak, and the subgenual cingulate becomes overactive, said Keith Sudheimer,

Ph.D., clinical assistant professor of psychiatry and a senior author of the study. Stimulating the subregion of the dorsolateral prefrontal cortex simultaneously reduces activity in the subgenual cingulate. One month after TMS therapy, 60% of participants were still in remission from depression. Follow-up studies are underway to determine the duration of the antidepressant effects. To test safety, the researchers evaluated the participants' cognitive function before and after treatment. They found no negative side effects; in fact, they discovered that the participants' ability to switch between mental tasks and to solve problems had improved — a typical outcome for people who are no longer depressed. [84]

---

[84] 2020. [online] Available at: <http://med.stanford.edu/news/all-news/2020/04/stanford-researchers-devise-treatment-that-relieved-depression-i.html> [Accessed 3 May 2020].

In 2019, a review study of hundreds of scientific studies regarding Brain Health entitled "Lifestyle Choices and Brain Health", AARP's Global Council on Brain Health concluded in its comprehensive study the importance of mental well-being, reporting that the restoration of brain health and mental well-being could potentially be a protective factor in the onset of any future neurodegenerative disorders later in life. The recommendations included within this study also echo Harvard Medical School's recommendations for optimization of brain health with emphasis on exercise, cognitively stimulating activities, sleep, nutrition, and social connectedness, [85] reminding us once again of the multi-dimensional nature of boosting brain health, including the utilization of

---

[85] 2020. [online] Available at: <https://www.ncbi.nlm.nih.gov/pmc/articles/PMC6787147/> [Accessed 4 May 2020].

neurostimulation and neurostimulating activities that ultimately induce Neuroplasticity and increased cerebral blood flow for brain optimization. Attention paid towards maintaining a balance aross all 8 major areas of life concurrently, as much as possible, will help you to acquire the sort of premium, satisfying, long-term improvements in brain health and in life that we all strive and hope for. Neurostimulation technologies as discussed in this book have been shown to be extremely capable for opening up new dimensions of health and performance capabilities through inducing neuroplasticity, increasing natural healing mechanisms such as stem cell growth, mitochondrial cell growth, and increasing cerebral blood flow. However, it is ultimately up to the individual to want to have these said benefits incorporated into their life. As with many health and performance modalities and technologies that , there exists the need for consistent utilization, embracing the routine practice of neurostimulation, for the benefits can certainly fade away over time, unfortunately.

TMS use studied for our four-legged pals

TMS therapy was performed on an in a 5-year-old neutered male Belgian Malinois dog showing anxious aggressive behavior in a 2019 study was published in the *Journal of Veterinary Behavior*. The research study used accelerated high-frequency repetitive transcranial magnetic stimulation (rTMS) which was proven to produce fast clinical effects in humans suffering from psychiatric illnesses as well. Although dogs also frequently present behavioral symptoms similar to mental illness, rTMS treatment was not yet investigated in canines. The aim of this study was to apply an rTMS treatment over the frontal cortex in an overly anxious and aggressive canine. Because rTMS is used to treat anxiety and mood disorders in humans and showed scientifically documented positive changes in neuronal activity and on monoamine concentrations, it was hypothesized that the dog's behavior would improve too after such a treatment. This improvement was expected to be accompanied by alterations in regional cerebral blood flow (rCBF). The researchers concluded that this research study demonstrated that a single day TMS treatment had indeed reduced the dog's overly anxious and aggressive behavior. This behavioral change was accompanied by immediate and long-lasting alterations in the cerebral blood flow (rCBF). This study confirms the interaction between the frontal cortex and the subcortical region of the canine's brain in regards to anxious types of behavior. The overly aggressive Belgian Melanois treated with TMS showed a corresponding decrease in aggression, an improvement in behavior that is attributed to increased cerebral blood flow. [86]

The Spirit of TMS

In the realm of minds, where echoes of storms reside, a gentle symphony of hope unfolds—a dance of transcranial magnetic stimulation therapy, an artistry of healing's touch.

Within the sacred chamber of the brain, a magnetic current weaves its magic, like a silken thread of light, tracing pathways through the labyrinth of thoughts. In the depths of neurons, it whispers tales of renewal, caressing the soul's untamed whispers.

---

[86] 2020. [online] Available at: <https://www.sciencedirect.com/science/article/abs/pii/S1558787818302284> [Accessed 22 May 2020].

Oh, how the magnetic waves dance, like fireflies on a moonlit night, illuminating the darkness of despair. With each tender pulse, they paint a masterpiece of healing upon the canvas of the mind, unraveling knots of pain with threads of resilience.

In the quiet sanctuary of the therapy's embrace, time slows its relentless march. Here, the heart's symphony finds harmony, and the soul finds solace in the sanctuary of restoration.

As the magnetic tides ebb and flow, they awaken dormant dreams, breathing life into the buried embers of hope. In the crucible of vulnerability, wounds find solace, for the therapy's touch knows no judgment or restraint.

In the gentle hum of the magnetic symphony, even the deepest wounds find liberation—their echoes diminishing, replaced by melodies of courage and renewal. Through the ethereal dance, the spirit's resilience takes flight, soaring beyond the limits of pain and affliction.

In the embrace of transcranial magnetic stimulation therapy, the mind becomes a canvas for transformation, and the heart becomes an instrument of healing's touch. It is a symphony of rebirth, an ode to the boundless human spirit.

So, let the magnetic waves cradle you, like a lullaby for the restless soul. Let it be the guiding light through the darkest nights, illuminating the path to restoration and renewal.

In the realm of minds, where echoes of storms once prevailed, a gentle symphony of hope unfolds—a dance of transcranial magnetic stimulation therapy, an artistry of healing's touch.

FAQs

Transcranial Magnetic Stimulation (TMS) therapy is a cutting-edge medical treatment that utilizes magnetic fields to stimulate specific regions of the brain. This non-invasive and painless procedure has shown promise in treating various mental health conditions and has become a beacon of hope for individuals seeking alternative therapies.

What is Transcranial Magnetic Stimulation (TMS) Therapy?

Transcranial Magnetic Stimulation (TMS) therapy is a form of brain stimulation that involves delivering magnetic pulses to targeted areas of the brain. These magnetic pulses are generated by a coil placed near the patient's scalp. The coil produces brief and focused magnetic fields that penetrate the skull and stimulate neurons in the brain.

How Does Transcranial Magnetic Stimulation Work?

During a TMS session, the magnetic pulses create small electrical currents in the brain, activating or modulating neural activity in the targeted area. This modulation can lead to changes in brain circuitry and the release of neurotransmitters, which are chemicals that facilitate communication between brain cells.

By stimulating specific brain regions, TMS can potentially alleviate symptoms associated with certain mental health disorders and promote neuroplasticity, the brain's ability to reorganize and form new connections.

Applications of Transcranial Magnetic Stimulation Therapy

Major Depressive Disorder (MDD)

TMS therapy has gained significant recognition as an effective treatment for Major Depressive Disorder (MDD), especially for patients who have not responded well to traditional antidepressant medications. By targeting the prefrontal cortex, which is involved in mood regulation, TMS can help improve symptoms of depression and enhance overall well-being.

Anxiety Disorders

Anxiety disorders, such as generalized anxiety disorder and social anxiety disorder, may also respond positively to TMS therapy. By influencing brain regions associated with anxiety, TMS can help reduce excessive worry, fear, and intrusive thoughts.

Post-Traumatic Stress Disorder (PTSD)

TMS has shown potential in the treatment of Post-Traumatic Stress Disorder (PTSD). By targeting brain areas involved in fear processing and emotional regulation, TMS can help individuals better manage traumatic memories and emotions associated with PTSD.

Obsessive-Compulsive Disorder (OCD)

For individuals with treatment-resistant OCD, TMS therapy can be a promising option. By stimulating brain regions linked to OCD symptoms, TMS may help reduce the severity of obsessions and compulsions.

Chronic Pain

TMS therapy has been investigated as a potential treatment for chronic pain conditions, such as fibromyalgia and neuropathic pain. By modulating pain pathways in the brain, TMS may provide relief and improve quality of life for individuals living with chronic pain.

Neurological Conditions

Research is ongoing to explore the applications of TMS in various neurological conditions, including epilepsy, Parkinson's disease, and multiple sclerosis. Although the field is still evolving, TMS shows potential as a complementary therapy in managing these conditions.

The TMS Procedure: What to Expect

A typical TMS session is performed in a clinical setting by trained healthcare professionals. The patient sits in a comfortable chair, and a specialized magnetic coil is positioned on their scalp over the target brain area. The coil is then activated, and the patient may feel a tapping or tingling sensation on their scalp during the magnetic pulses.

TMS sessions are generally well-tolerated and do not require anesthesia, allowing patients to remain awake and alert throughout the procedure. The duration and frequency of TMS sessions may vary depending on the individual's condition and treatment plan.

Is Transcranial Magnetic Stimulation Safe?

Transcranial Magnetic Stimulation therapy is considered safe when administered by qualified professionals. It is non-invasive and does not require surgery or the use of anesthesia. Side effects are generally mild and transient, with the most common being temporary scalp discomfort and headaches.

As with any medical treatment, it's essential for patients to discuss their medical history and any potential contraindications with their healthcare provider before starting TMS therapy.

How long does a typical TMS session last?

A standard TMS session usually lasts around 20 to 30 minutes. However, the duration may vary depending on the specific treatment protocol and individual needs.

How many TMS sessions are typically required for depression treatment?

The number of TMS sessions needed for depression treatment can vary depending on the individual's response and the severity of the condition. Generally, a course of treatment consists of multiple sessions over several weeks.

Is TMS covered by health insurance?

TMS therapy may be covered by some health insurance plans, especially for specific mental health conditions and when other treatments have been ineffective. Patients are advised to check with their insurance providers for coverage details.

Can TMS be combined with other therapies?

Yes, TMS therapy can be combined with other treatments, such as psychotherapy or medication, to enhance overall treatment outcomes. It's essential to work with healthcare providers to develop a comprehensive treatment plan.

Does TMS have any long-term effects on the brain?

Research suggests that TMS therapy does not cause any long-term adverse effects on brain structure or function. It is considered a safe and well-tolerated treatment option for mental health disorders.

Conclusion

Transcranial Magnetic Stimulation (TMS) therapy represents a promising frontier in the field of mental health and neuroscience. By harnessing the power of magnetic fields to influence brain activity, TMS offers new possibilities for treating depression, anxiety, and other mental health disorders. As research and understanding of this innovative therapy continue to evolve, TMS has the potential to transform the landscape of mental health treatments and provide hope to those in need.

Notes Section for Action Steps